Ask Ed

Marijuana Success

Ask Ed: Marijuana Success — Grow Cannabis Year-Round
by Ed Rosenthal

Copyright © 2020 Ed Rosenthal
Published by Quick American
A Division of Quick Trading Co.
Piedmont, CA, USA

ISBN: 9781936807499
eISBN: 9781936807505

Printed in the United States
First Printing

Editor and Project Manager: Rolph Blythe
Art Director: Christian Petke
Design: Scott Idleman / Blink
Cover Design: Christian Petke

Cover Photography: Lizzy Cozzi

Library of Congress Number: 2018953922

Ask Ed

Marijuana Success

Grow Cannabis Year-Round

by Ed Rosenthal

ACKNOWLOWLEDGMENTS

Rolph Blythe, Boveda, Rebecca Chambers, Julie Chiariello, Good Earth Organics, Green Pad, Chris Grunenberg, Harvest-More, Humboldt Seed Company, Jane Klein, Paradise Seeds, Christian Petke, Gopi Lennon, Brian Lundeen, Ryan Miller, Purple Caper Seeds, Relic Seeds, Sensi Seeds, Smart Pots Subcool, Marisa Sympson, Darcy Thompson, Tom's Tumble Trimmer, Seed Cellar

RUN FOR THE ROSES

Man, oh, man, oh, friend of mine
All good things in all good time
Reach for the sun, catch hold of the moon
They're both too heavy but what can you do?
Reach for the stars, smack into the sky

Run, run, run for the roses

—Jerry Garcia/Robert Hunter
Courtesy of the Grateful Dead

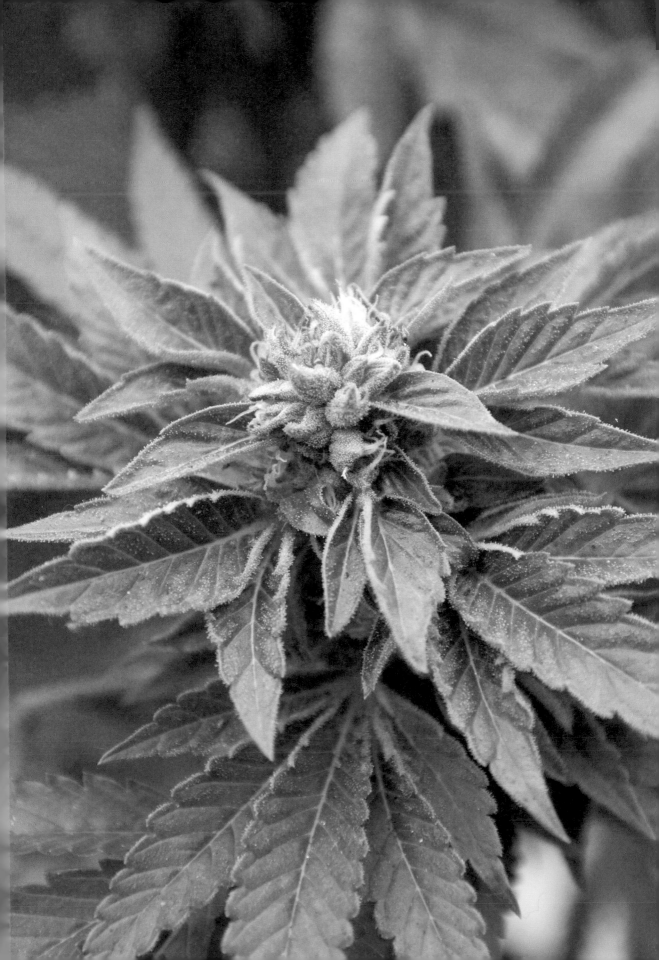

Table of Contents

VARIETIES

1. Testing the Varieties: Which Strain is Right for You? **10**

- How to test many varieties' growth and potency
- Growing many plants in a small space

2. Cultivar Bazar: High Quality Strains for Hobbyists **20**

TIPS TO INCREASE EFFICIENCY

3. Lessons from a Hawaiian Garden **28**

- Outdoors: Extending the Light Period to Keep Plants Growing Vegetatively

4. Hawaiian Legal **34**

- Indoors: Extending light period for vegetating

5. Lessons from a Jamaica Winter Garden **38**

- Growing in a short-day environment using close planting

6. Plant Regeneration: How to Achieve a Second Harvest . . . **42**

7. Tweaking Bud Potency Using UV Light **44**

8. Summer Interlude: Wick System in my Greenhouse **48**

- The low-water, easy-to-care-for wick system
- Manicuring & drying

9. Building Wick Systems **52**

- The most environmentally friendly setup

10. The Benefits of Small Plants **56**

11. Cannabis Seeds or Clones: Which is Right for You? **60**

12. Your Essential Guide to When Cannabis Buds Are Ready to Harvest . . . **64**

GROWING WITH THE SEASONS

13. California Winter Garden **70**

- Starting clones in a greenhouse
- How to have a successful spring harvest

14. Fall Quickie Garden **80**

- How to plant late in the season for a fall harvest

15. Winter Garden **84**

- Using natural and supplemental light
- Growing with the changing seasons

16. A Three-Month Spring/Summer Garden **88**

- Planting to maximize light
- Mobile gardens
- Outdoors or in a greenhouse? Both!

17. Ask Ed: Common Drying and Harvesting Questions **98**

18. Garden Fever **104**

- Exploring different hydroponic methods
- Simple light deprivation methods to speed up ripening

GOING COMMERCIAL

19. Ketama: Morocco's Cannabis Paradise **114**

- Traditional use of tight planting for greater yield

20. Inside Kind Love's Marijuana Production Facility **118**

- Professional cloning techniques
- Air circulation techniques
- Tips for increasing efficiency at home or in a commercial garden

21. Ask Ed: Common Lighting Questions **122**

22. Oakland Garden: Is This the Largest Urban Grow in the United States? . . **124**

Large scale container growing
- SOP (Standard Operating Procedure) of harvest

RAINY DAY CRAFT

23. Hashimals: Enjoying the End Product **134**

24. Ask Ed: Pot-Pourri—A Final Selection of Questions from Readers . . . **138**

Sponsors **140**

Introduction

By Ed Rosenthal

You will find between these covers a journal of my home garden experiments as well as cultivations I visited here and abroad.

I use my small garden to test new methods of cultivation, so this book provides a lot of thought-provoking information about growing marijuana. There's a little something for everyone here: from growing seasonally to working with soil, hydro systems, plants of all sizes, harvesting, drying and curing.

Although the gardens are small, the cultivation techniques can be up-scaled to much larger sites. The reason: The techniques are about the plants, not plumbing or electrical circuitry.

Even if you have been growing for a while, I think you will find this an interesting read, containing proven methods you might not be familiar with. These methods are sure to save you time, money and labor.

A grower friend read the manuscript and said, "Before I read this I didn't know what I didn't know. Very helpful."

Exactly!

Ed

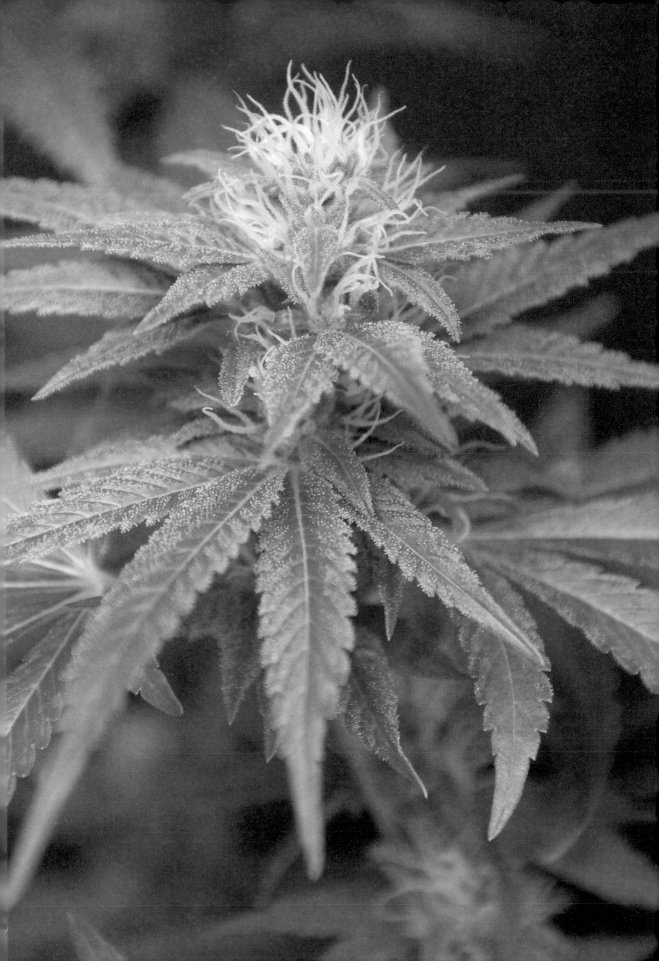

Chapter 1

Testing the Varieties
WHICH STRAIN IS RIGHT FOR YOU?

Covers:
- How to test many varieties' growth and potency
- Growing many plants in a small space

As a consumer, you might have some experience with strains like Gorilla Glue and OG Kush. If not, it's easy enough to look at their stats and read some reviews before purchasing for consumption, or you can buy grams of each and compare the medicines yourself.

It's a little different when choosing varieties to grow. I live in an area with many dispensaries that sell clones. They have a huge selection of varieties, between ten and fifty in each shop. So there are hundreds of varieties to choose from.

When deciding on new varieties to grow either for personal use or for distribution, there will be new sets of concerns. What's the plant's branching habit? How much does it grow after forcing? What's the time until ripening? Which varieties do best under the methods you use? What are the strains' comparative yields?

A plant trial can answer such questions. The method I'm designing is a template and a model for testing. With the proliferation of hybrids and varieties, plant trials are essential for growers to determine what they plan to grow. Other trials may be used

- to choose the best progeny from propagated seeds.
- to test the effect of new cultivation practices on the varieties being grown.
- to choose the best plant to clone from purchased seeds.
- to test different cultivation practices.
- to test different fertilizers and fertilizer regimens.

WHEN ALL ELSE FAILS, CONDUCT AN EXPERIMENT

The purpose of this testing model is to minimize time, labor, energy, and space, making it feasible for ordinary gardeners, small and large, to run a relatively extensive test fairly easily.

In this case I used miniature plants of each variety to replicate how a particular strain might perform if it had more space and time to develop into a larger plant. To do this, I forced the plants to flower when they were still small, only 10 days after they had been transplanted into 6-inch containers.

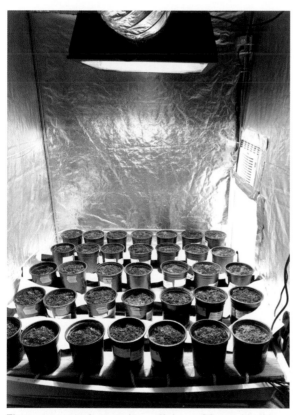

The tent was ready to go. It was lit by an OG metal halide 860-watt and has AC, CO_2, air circulation a hybrid planting mix/hydro system.

THE DESIGN

The experiment was conducted in a $5' \times 5'$ garden tent. It has a vertical hanging metal halide 860-watt lamp in a sophisticated air-cooled reflector that limits the heat released into the garden. The light was controlled by a timer.

Excess heat was controlled using a small recirculating air conditioner installed in the sidewall that sits on a table outside.

The air was enriched with CO_2 using a 20-pound tank regulated by a sensor set to keep the space at 1200 parts per million (ppm) during the lit hours.

A small oscillating fan keeps the air in the space circulating continuously.

A recording thermometer that shows the high and low temperature was hung from the tubing so that it was at canopy level. The temperature controller was set never to go below 60 degrees.

The plants were put in two 1-quart, 6-inch containers filled with a mixture of 50% coir and about 25% each homemade aged compost (derived from plant leaf, fruit drop, and food waste) plus some planting mix left over from previous projects.

A double-ended, ⅜-inch braided nylon wick extended from either end of the opposite-facing holes at the bottom of the container. The ends trailed into the tray below. To prevent fraying, the wick was tied using twist ties.

The thirty-five containers sat on a wooden pallet placed inside a $4' \times 4'$ tray filled with rainwater that had been pH'd to 6.0. A one-part complete hydroponic vegetative formula 7-9-5 with potassium silicate had been added to the water at 700 ppm.

The water was circulated in the tray using two small water pumps, each pushing about 600 gallons per hour. It was aerated using four airstones powered by a small aquarium pump. An aquarium heater rated for 40 gallons kept the water at 70 degrees. The tray sat on a piece of ½-inch-thick Styrofoam that created a barrier between it and the cold cement floor.

GETTING THE GARDEN GOING

If you want to try this experiment in your garden, follow this process:

1. Label each plant using a plastic marker placed in the container and an additional identifying tag attached to the stem. Mark them with a soft pencil (3, 4B, H, or 2H). Ink often fades.

2. Place the seedlings or clones in the containers. The stem should not be deeper than it is when you start. If need be, use a skewer or other support to keep the stem upright. Use a high-quality planting mix.

3. Water after potting with diluted vegetative-stage fertilizer water (400 ppm). This is one of the few times you'll do this. In the future the planting mix will draw water/nutrient solution up the nylon wick, as needed.

4. Set the light on continuously for seven to ten days or up to thirty days for seedlings. Then turn the light off for a day to spur the plants to transition from growing vegetatively to flowering.

5. The NEXT DAY turn the light back on, but use a timer so the space receives 12 hours of light and 12 hours of total darkness daily.

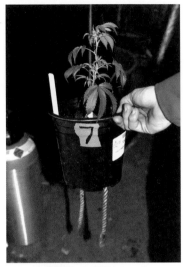

Each of the 35 plants is in a 6" container with a wick that draws water up using capillary action.

6. Keep this light-dark regimen for the next month. During the dark period the plants require UNINTERRUPTED darkness. Do not open the curtain or door or turn on the lights during the dark period, even for a moment. The only light that can be safely used during the dark period is laser or LED green.

7. Fertilize with a vegetative formula such as 7-9-5 at 700 ppm. Adjust the pH in the water using pH up or pH down to 5.6–6.2.

8. At the same time you change the flowering cycle, change the fertilizer to flowering stage formula, which is low in nitrogen and high in phosphorous and potassium. You don't have to drain the try. Just add new water to it as needed.

9. Make sure the heater doesn't blow or radiate directly on the leaves. During the lit period the ideal leaf temperature

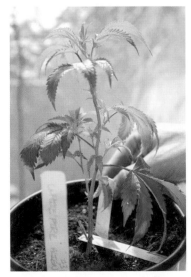

Each plant is tagged twice- in the container and on the stem. Use a pencil because inks run and fade.

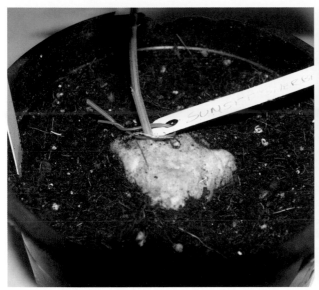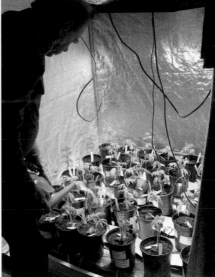

Plants were placed in their new containers keeping the stem at the same depth it was in the starter cube. The plants are being watered with diluted nutrient/water solution with beneficial mycorrhizae added. This helps the cube make close contact and settle in the mix.

is about 85 degrees. Use a surface temperature thermometer to check leaf temperature. Then adjust the AC and heater to keep the leaf temperature between 80 and 85 degrees. During the dark period the temperature should not fall below 60 degrees, but it's best kept above 70 to inhibit fungal infections. Use a heater to raise the temperature if needed.

ALWAYS CHECK YOUR PLANTING MIX

I had prepared the soil using fibrous and chunky coir, previously used planting mix, and homemade compost. As soon as the plants came in contact with the mix, they began showing symptoms of various nutrient problems, including calcium (Ca), magnesium (Mg), and iron (Fe) deficiencies as well as unidentified fertilizer burn.

At first I thought it was only a Ca/Mg deficiency, which sometimes occurs even in fertilized water here in the San Francisco Bay Area, because of the low natural mineral content. This is common in water derived from snow runoff, the East Bay's water source. I decided to add extra Ca and Mg to the water using a fertilizer composed of the two minerals. This solved some of the problems, but there were still signs of overfertilization as well as Fe deficiency.

Plant list
- Ghost OG
- Blue Dream
- Dream Queen
- Pruple Urkle
- AC-DC
- White fire Alien
- OG GDP
- Sunset Sherbet
- THC Bond
- GSC
- Mendo Kush
- Kosher Kush
- Gorilla Glue
- Dead Head
- Gorilla Blue #4
- Larry OG
- Candyland
- Platinum Purple

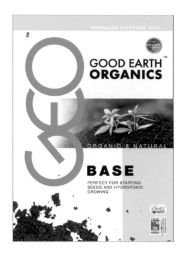 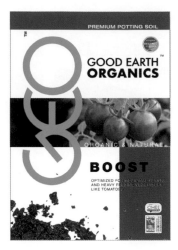 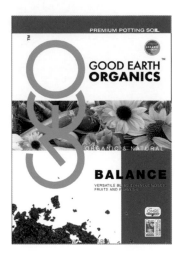

Good Earth Organics (GEO) offers a full line of soils and nutrients optimized for cannabis. All Good Earth Organics soils are approved for organic growing; they are OMRI approved and Clean Green Certified. Good Earth Organics soils and nutrients work as a system to provide the right soil environment and nutrient support for strong yields and "pure" quality. Good Earth Organics soils are carefully blended from high quality components to ensure consistency so growers can expect consistent results. GEO soils can be reused for up to three harvests.

Analyzing the symptoms further, I realized that the planting mix was the cause of the problems. The coir had been washed before it was used, so I didn't think that it contained excess salts from the manufacturing process. Other plants were growing in combinations of my aged used planting mix, so that wasn't the problem. That left the homemade compost. It had been slow aged for over a year and was crumbly with a healthy earthy odor. However, it was probably absorbing some nutrients and releasing too concentrated a mix of others, preventing the plants from getting proper nutrition.

The solution: I ran nutrient water solution through the containers three times over the next few days. This provided extra nutrients lacking in the   planting mix so that the plants would absorb as much as they could use. At the same time, the overconcentrated nutrients were rinsed away. The roots were immediately able to absorb nutrients directly from the water. Within days the new growth showed signs of total recovery.

I decided to move the plants to a larger space because they were growing more vigorously than I anticipated, even though they were flowering. I removed them from the grow tent, and the thirty-five plants were placed in a 4′ × 8′ tray in a greenhouse, giving them just a little less than a square foot per plant to finish flowering. Right now they are getting natural light enhanced with 8 hours of a 1000-watt HPS lamp on a track.

Nutrient Problem Symptoms:

- Ca deficiency: necrosis of edges and then interior of new as well as older leaves. It appears as brown dried spots.
- Mg deficiency: leaves in the middle first and then in upper leaves as well; the veins remain green while the tissue in-between turns yellow.
- Fe deficiency: upper leaves grow bright pale yellow.
- Fertilizer burn: leaves curl down or up, sometimes look ultra-dark green.

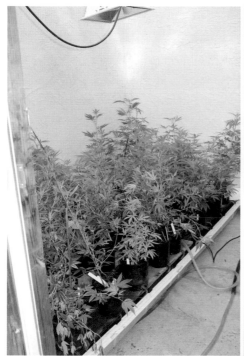

The garden a month from beginning flowering.

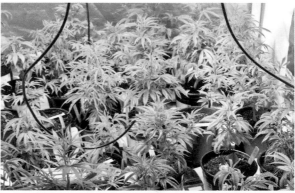

THC Bomb one week after the light period was reduced. Notice that the plant was suffering from nutrient deficiencies.

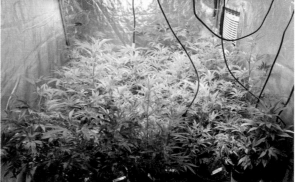

The garden two weeks later.

DELAYS, DELAYS, DELAYS

About halfway through flowering, the process slowed, delaying ripening for a few weeks. There were several reasons.

First, the Bay Area has had weeks of mostly cloudy or rainy weather, limiting the amount of light the plants received as compared with what they receive on sunny days, even in the low-light months of February and March. Second, about three weeks into flowering, the lighting schedule suffered from a malfunctioning timer. The plants received 2 to 4 extra hours of light each day for five days. This probably delayed ripening by ten to twelve days.

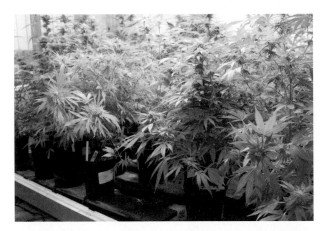

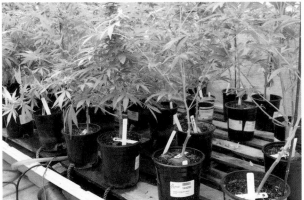

The greenhouse receives light only from the top and the front. The other sides are building walls. To supplement the natural light, two 1000-watt HPS lamps switch on from 10 a.m. to 4 p.m. One is on a light mover and the other is attached to the back wall to light the darker back part of the greenhouse.

Since the plants are close to one another, their sides and understory leaves and branches don't get much light. Light powers both the plant's growth and its metabolism, so these parts don't contribute to the plant's growth. Instead, they use energy produced by the canopy to fuel their metabolism, and they hinder the free flow of air between the plants. Removing them eases crowding, facilitates airflow, and lessens the energy load that nonproductive parts use.

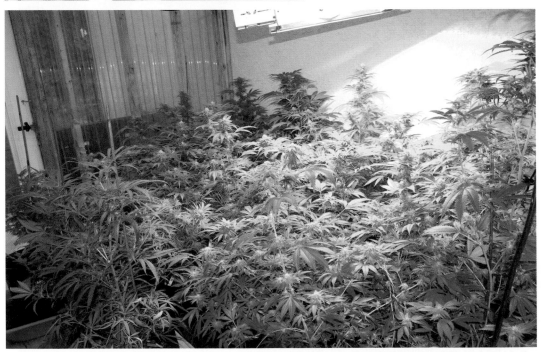

1. The plants in the garden before pruning away the lower branches. 2. After pruning the air flows freely and the plants have a bit more space. 3. The greenhouse. Besides the 35 experimental plants 6 plants that were living outdoors to get an early start on the summer have taken up temporary residence to stay out of the rain.

HARVEST AND DRYING

This was a winter garden, and it was before the vernal equinox (March 22), so the plants received fewer than 12 hours of light. The garden harvest began on March 25, just six weeks after the plants were placed into flowering. All of them ripened within two weeks. Once they were cut, some of the fan leaves were removed, and the plants were hung to dry in a cool room.

Usually the drying room stays between 65 and 70 degrees, but it's been cool recently, and the room temperature has stayed in the low 60s, which slows drying. It's also been cloudy and rainy, keeping the average relative humidity around 65%. Fifty percent is ideal for drying and curing. So after two weeks the plants were still a little moist, very pliable, and not ready to take the next step in their journey, manicuring.

To speed things up, I plugged in a dehumidifier that heated the room a little bit and removed moisture.

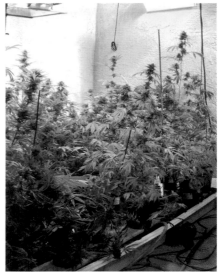

The 35 plants in the greenhouse are ready to harvest.

Learning from the Shape of Your Plants

The plants had different shapes while growing. As they hang without fan leaves, it's easy to see the shapes that the plants developed. Before removing the buds, I photographed each plant. The buds were manicured and then weighed and tested for cannabinoid content. This provided a profile of their relative yield and their shape.

Having this information can help growers plan their gardens or fields, for example, how far apart to space the plants and how to prune them for bigger yields.

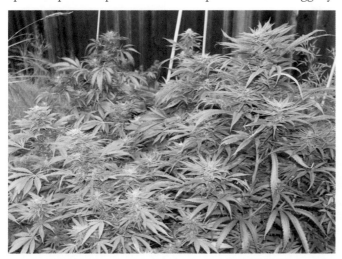

Six of the plants spent most of their flowering time outdoors.

When this experiment was first started, I ended up with some extra clones that I eventually planted in 3-gallon containers. I placed the plants outside and let them go. Five of the six plants ripened about a week after the last greenhouse plants were harvested. So those plants were cut, leaving only small, immature buds and leaves from the lower part of the plant.

The THC levels were not high. The main reason is that the plants were receiving only a mod-

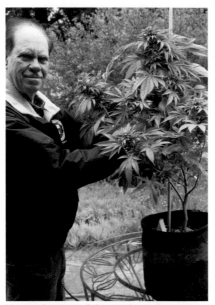

Harvesting one of the outdoor plants.

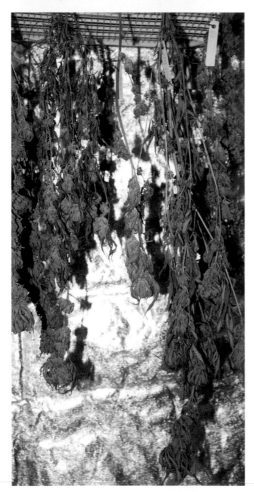

Here's how the varieties tested in THC order:

Customer sample name	Heated THC	Heated CBD
Blueberry 46	18.7285	←1.5
Tahoe OG /44	18.5799	←1.5
THC bomb /40	17.8746	←1.5
Sunset Sherbert	17.0002	←1.5
Fire OG /11	16.4761	←1.5
Candyland /21	16.3428	←1.5
Ghost OG /38	16.3067	←1.5
Purple cream/29	16.1856	←1.5
Headband /47	16.1766	←1.5
Deadhead OG/34	16.0319	←1.5
Larry OG /33	15.6465	←1.5
Double Dream	15.4269	←1.5
GDP/19	15.3888	←1.5
Sour D	15.2815	←1.5
xj/13/1	14.9222	←1.5
LA fire/26	14.7357	←1.5
Blue Dream /39	14.7292	←1.5
Dream Queen/18	14.4515	←1.5
Kosher Kush	13.6575	←1.5
Pure OG Kush	13.6575	←1.5
Gorilla glue/10	13.4882	←1.5
Purple Diesel/24	12.3195	←1.5
Harlequin GDP/50	7.3913	8.33525
Harlequin/57	6.05688	7.38588
ACDC /43,	←2	10.4476
ACDC /43	←2	10.5485

erate amount of light during flowering. The total amount of light averaged only about 10.5 hours daily. The winter and early spring sunlight received was weak and mostly indirect. Even supplemented with 6 hours of HPS light, this was still too little to produce maximum bud development and to reach THC potential.

The differences in THC levels show the relative THC/CBD potentials of the varieties. Notice how many varieties placed in the 16% to 14% range. Except for specialty varieties, all had virtually no CBD. Varieties differ in effects because they have different ratios of terpenes, odor molecules that affect mood and have medical qualities.

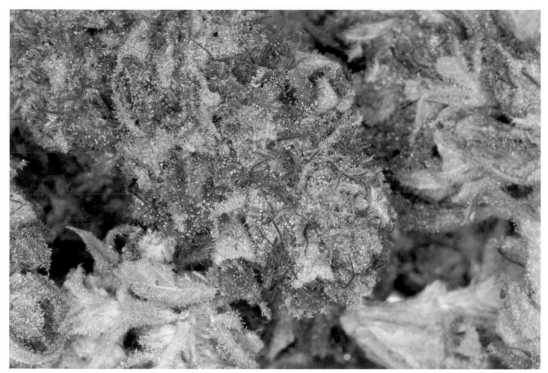

Close-up of dried Harlequin Bud

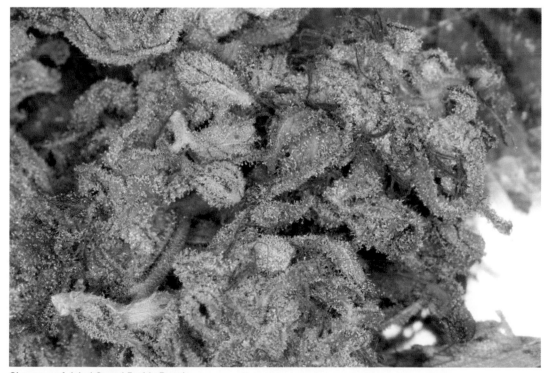

Close-up of dried Grand Daddy Purple

Chapter 2

Cultivar Bazaar:
High quality strains for hobbyists

I asked some of my favorite seed breeders to suggest their best cultivar for home growers. The stipulations were that each was easy to grow, adapted easily to different environments, and most importantly, that it had a distinctive personality. The breeders responded with some great suggestions.

Each cultivar is handsome, above average and potently effective. A garden featuring these selections will provide you with a library of wonderful sensations to fit time, space and mood. A couple of the strains produce high ratios of CBD.

Here's the list.:

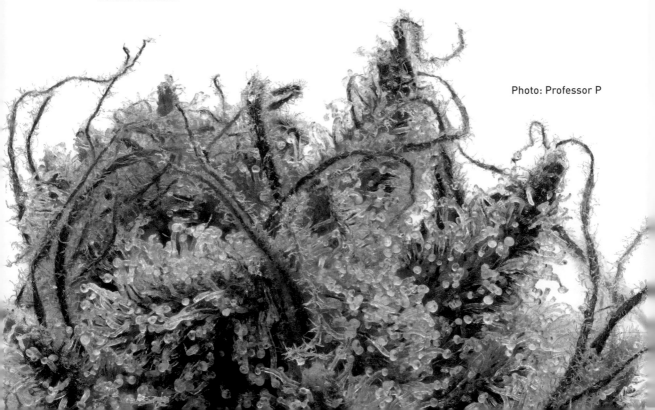

Photo: Professor P

Blueberry Muffin

Parents: The Razz (Razzleberry) x P.P.D. (formerly known as Purple Panty Dropper

Indica/Sativa ratio: 65% - 35%

Breeder: Nathaniel Pennington

Seed Company: Humboldt Seed Company

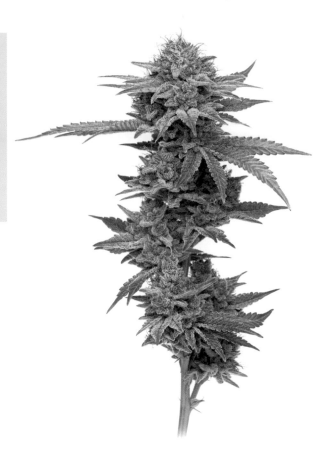

Humboldt Seeds recommends Blueberry Muffin because it is easy to grow. It has a sturdy stalk and resistance to molds, mildews and pests. This strain pretty much maintains itself.

Blueberry Muffin is a shorter stocky type 65%-35% Indica/Sativa hybrid that produces bountiful buds for its size, beautifully tinged with purple flakes. With a quick flowering cycle of 45-60 days you will have plump, trichome coated buds before you know it.

The variety grows well both indoors and outdoors, but it tends to stretch unless it is pruned to branch. Once pruned, it can be trained to a screen of green (scrog).

Both environments bring out the real blueberry muffin smell that has been compared favorably to the Jiffy brand Blueberry Muffin Mix. The fruity aroma extends to the flavor of the inhalation. Leafly reviews show Blueberry Muffin is the world's most aptly named strain. Some heads up for indoor growers: Be prepared for pervasive terpenes that tend to overpower any other varietals in a grow room or greenhouse.

Blueberry Muffin is also known for the fact that it seems to lack any paranoia inducing characteristics. The high is relaxing and happy and induces a positive attitude. It can be used when doing routine work, but it does not encourage creativity or mind wandering. This is useful for medical patients medicating throughout the day. It's also a good choice for individuals new to cannabis.

"Blueberry Muffin is a gentle strain that is here on this earth to help people... she wants to be given organic soil and real sun ideally, but she will provide her medicine whenever and however she is needed" —Humboldt Seed Company

Cheese Quake—For both indoor and outdoor gardens
Parents: Exodus Cheese X Querkle (Urkle x Space Queen)
Indica/Sativa ratio: 60% - 40%
Breeder: Subcool
Seed Company: The Dank

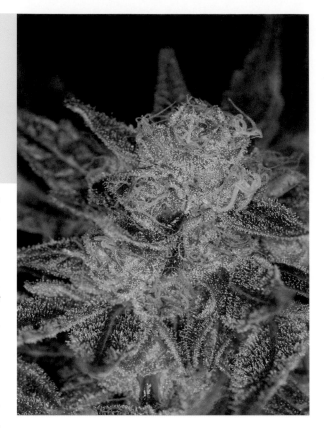

When asked about a recommendation for home-growers, Subcool enthusiastically recommends Cheese Quake "It's easy to grow and pretty to look at."

It's a heavy producer with purple leaves and an aroma that is a blend of fruit and cheese, which it inherited from its parents Querkle and Cheese. The buds are more round than cone shape. Cheese Quake grows well both indoors and outdoors. Indoors the plant is short and stocky. Outdoors, it grows over 6 ft tall given enough time without being topped. This variety is perfect for SOG when it is flowered early. Flowering time is 8-9 weeks.

The terpene profile is high in Myrcene, which enables the high to take effect sooner because of its ability to allow THC to reach the brain cells more rapidly. Even Subcool has been surprised at the intensity of the high. He describes it as "mental energy that can be confusing, yet delightful." However, in reviews two thirds of respondents used the terms, happy, relaxed, and euphoric Myrcene is also associated with analgesic and anti-depressive qualities. Reviewers also noted relief from stress and anxiety as well as muscular pain.

Subcool describes the taste as a "Grape Cheese Danish." It picks up the grape from the Querkle on the inhale and an exhale that is the cherry and the sourness associated with the cheese varieties.

"By combining the grapey-lavender taste of Purple Urkle with the unique smell and taste of Cheese created a flavor so incredible it instantly became my favorite Cheese hybrid."
—Subcool.

Mendocino Skunk

Parents: Skunk #1, Haze, and Afghani
Indica/Sativa ratio: 60% - 40%
Breeder's Name: Luc Krol
Seed Company Name: Paradise Seeds

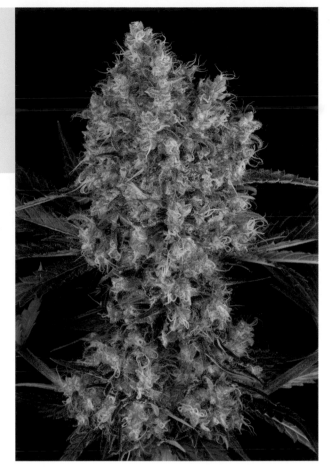

When asked to recommend a variety for the hobby grower Mendocino Skunk was the clear choice. It's part of the Tommy Chong collection.

Mendocino Skunk is a very manageable plant because it does not get too large, accommodating growers with limited growing space. Size does not limit the yield. The plant is short, with a thick central cola and robust side branches. Indoors the plant grows up to 5 feet. Outdoors, especially in sunny climates and given enough time, the plant grows to 6.5 feet tall. It has a higher flower to leaves ration and more dry weight than many classic Indica skunk strains

The Mendocino genetics make this a good choice for northern USA, Europe, and Canada Flowering time is 7-8 weeks.

In developing this hybrid Paradise Seeds created a high that balances the energizing qualities of Sativas with the relaxing effect of Indicas resulting in an experience generally described as positive and uplifting. Routine daily tasks can be handled as normal, and with even more focus. Myrcene, Caryophyllene, and Limonene are the dominant terpenes. And of course, there is that robust aroma of earthy skunkiness.

"It was a challenge for us when Tommy Chong asked us to develop seeds that are called Choice of Legends, but we worked hard in our breeding rooms and we are super pleased with the final results." —Paradise Seeds

Grapefruit Web

Parents: Charlotte's Web x Grapefruit Web F2
Indica/Sativa ratio: 60% - 40%
Breeder: Professor P
Seed Company: Relic Seeds

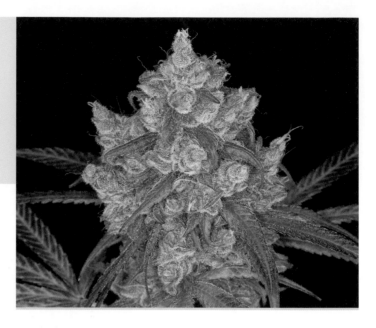

Relic Seeds' recommendation of Grapefruit Web is a variety that offers a balanced 1:1 ratio of CBD and THC. The Mom, Charlotte's Web is a legendary high CBD cultivar recognized for medicinal use. The Dad provided by SowLow Farms contributed a rich array of terpenes resulting in a very tasty hybrid.

Both parents passed down performance as high yielders to their progeny. Grapefruit Web is a beast of a plant, producing enormous colas of massive proportions. The breeder advises that stakes are certainly required considering the girth on the terminal buds.

The plant performs well indoors and out. Grapefruit Web grows in the typical Xmas tree shape with large spear shaped colas. There is a slight purple fade during maturation. Flowering time is shorter than average; 7-8 weeks.

Smelling like fresh cut pink grapefruit, the aroma and taste are refreshing, yet calming due to the terpene profile. The top four terpenes are beta-Myrcene, Linalool, Limonene and Pinene balancing the alertness induced by Pinene with the relaxation associated with Linalool.

Grapefruit Web has an extremely inviting buzz, great for users of all levels. It's an even keeled head/body high that is great for any time of the day. Described on Leafly as Happy and Uplifting this is a good flower to offset stress and anxiety.

"She's an easy plant to succeed with for several reasons: Easy to grow, large yields, and short bloom times" —Relic Seeds

Northern Lights

Parents: NL #1 x NL #2 x NL#3
Indica/Sativa ratio: 90% -10%
Breeder: Sensi Seeds
Seed Company: Sensi Seeds

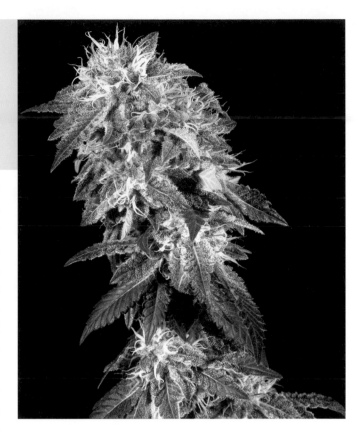

Northern Lights is a classic strain and one of the most famous Indica varieties. There are now many variations on its name and genetics. During its original development, Sensi Seeds was able to acquire one of three pure types of Northern Lights, and have maintained the intent of plant vigor and potency.

A petite plant averaging between 3½-5 feet, Northern Lights is fast-flowering, resilient, and produces dense, resin-rich flowers. Highly adapted to Indoor growing, Northern Lights is a satisfying yielder that can finish in just over 6 weeks. It is very well suited to the Sea of Green method. Because the buds are so dense, be sure to provide a proper airflow to prevent any humidity build-up within them. In cooler climate, it will give excellent results when grown in a greenhouse. In warmer climates Northern Lights will do well outdoors, developing into massive trees.

The aroma is pungently sweet herbal aroma with pepper and citrus notes and the taste is a flavorful mixture of sweet and spice.

Although Northern Lights is a high THC strain with very little CBD present, the presence of the terpenes Myrcene, Caryophyllene and Limonene result in a very calming effect. This strain is a great variety to relax and can be used to ease stress and pain. It is also well suited to people having issues sleeping.

"This strain is great one for beginners and experts alike and is available in regular, feminized and auto-flowering variants." —Sensi Seeds

Sensi Skunk

Parents: (Afghani x Skunk#1) x
Skunk#1
Indica/Sativa ratio: 80% - 20%
Breeder: Sensi Seeds
Seed Company: Sensi Seeds

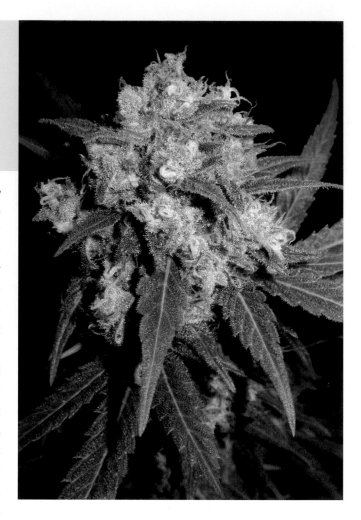

Sensi Skunk is a potent hybrid, leaning heavily towards Indica characteristics. The variety is a favorite with beginners and aficionados alike. Sensi Seeds specifically bred the variety for ease of cultivation. It has a vigorous growth pattern with a comparatively short flowering time.

The plant is average in height with strong branches, easily manageable growth, rapidly-swelling buds and sizeable harvest of thick, pungent colas covered in resin. Left to its own devices, this plant grows in a Christmas tree shape with a main central cola. The plant can produce a large yield with minimal care; it is easy to grow indoors and outdoors.

Outdoors this plant's potential is truly expressed, producing high yields between the end September and mid-October. In temperate climates Sensi Skunk grows well in a normal warm summer. The breeder recommends cultivating below 42 degrees north, which covers USA gardens from the Oregon-California border across to the NY-Pennsylvania border and south. This also includes Southern Europe, parts of China and even North Korea.

Sensi Skunk delivers an attention grabbing sugary-citrus bouquet that's uniquely different from the regular Skunk funk. A refreshing sweet-citrus aroma infuses each bud. The overall effect of Sensi Skunk is a balanced one. Its effects will make you relaxed, happy, and euphoric, without being overwhelmingly strong.

> "Quick to bloom, thick-budding and potent enough to surprise even a jaded smoker, Sensi Skunk is also very forgiving when growing and flowering, making her a strain that is actually quite difficult to mess up." —Sensi Seeds

Chocolate Tonic

Parents: Cannatonic x Chocolate Kush
Indica/Sativa: 35% - 65%
Seed Breeder: The Purple Caper
Seed Company: Purple Caper Seeds

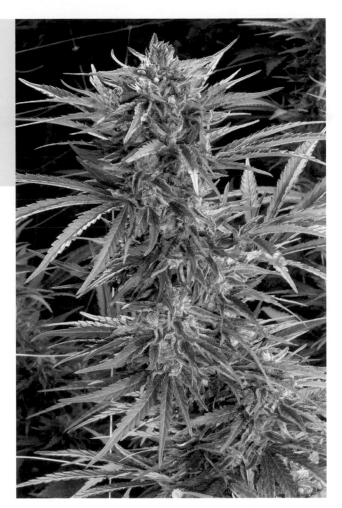

This strain originated from a CBD project designed to help patients with a range of conditions: pain management, seizures, and inflammation, and cancer treatment. The breeder crossed a high THC father with a high CBD mother. Both were chosen for their cannabinoid content, vigor, and yield, and the tendency to pass the desired traits from each to the offspring. Chocolate Tonic offers a 2:1 CBD to THC ratio. The typical gardener can expect 14% CBD and 7% THC, as well as small amounts of CBC and CBG.

Chocolate Tonic is very versatile and can grow in any environment. It takes on a Xmas tree shape with little branching so best to prune from above. Plants can reach heights of 8 feet outdoors. It's a strong grower that can withstand heat, drought, and even being root-bound. Outdoors, when planted in May and grown in the ground or planted with 6-foot centers, look for a yield of 3 pounds per plant. Ripens in October. Indoors flowering time is 8-10 weeks. Expect 1.5 pounds per light.

Pain relief is a key feature of the high. The numbing and relaxing qualities are also sleep inducing after a long day. Chocolate Tonic lives up to its name with a chocolate, piney, citrus flavor.

"This CBD strain grows like a weed and can handle abuse." —Purple Caper

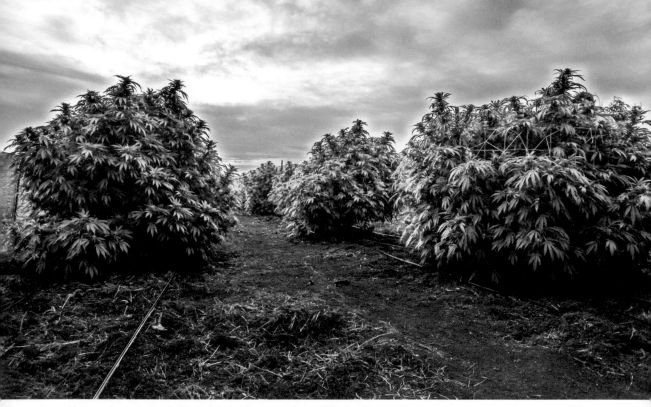

Mature plants in the field. Molokai skies have about 25% cloud cover. Even so, the plants receive intense light and plenty of UV spectrum.

Chapter 3

Lessons from a Hawaiian Garden

Covers:
- Outdoors: Extending the light period to keep plants glowing vegetatively

Hawaii is fabled for its fine marijuana. Anticipating the Hawaii Cannabis Expo in February, in Oahu, I expected to sample some fine entries. And I wasn't disappointed. The intense sun at the 21st latitude (for reference, Key West, Florida, is the 24th latitude), and the mild island weather creates great cultivation environments.

    I wasn't a judge, but I did try many of the varieties. The samples included several fine sativa and sativa-indica hybrids, which do especially well under the intense sun and are genetically inclined to resist flowering under short days. However, there was better to be had.

I was innocently hanging outside the Blaisdell Center, where the conference was held, and was invited to join a small circle of newfound friends. A fellow pulled out an extra-wide. I understood immediately that he was a successful grower who was confident in his product's quality.

The mildness of the draw, combined with the fine terpenes and high levels of THC and, I suspect, THCV, was a recipe for pleasure creation and key to mind-opening awareness and creativity. Proof that cannabis liberates the wandering mind, opening it to emotion, love, and beauty. This was certainly excellent weed. And good reason for Dustin's (one of my new friends) cheerful attitude.

Dustin invited us to come visit the island where he lived. We took his invitation seriously. In December we flew back to Hawaii and visited Molokai for the first time.

Until Hawaii legalized cultivation of medical marijuana, outdoor growing was policed heavily by law enforcement. Happily, after legalization, the gardens have moved to backyards and other domestic spaces.

Hawaii has a climate similar to some low-latitude areas of the United States such as Florida, portions of the Gulf Coast, and Southern California. They stay warm enough and get enough light to support plant growth throughout the year. The problem is dealing with day length. The closer a place is to the equator, the smaller the difference between summer-winter light-dark hours.

On June 21, the longest day of the year, there are 13 hours and 25 minutes of light. On December 21, the shortest day, there are 10 hours and 51 minutes of light. Marijuana is a short-day

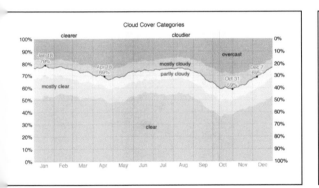

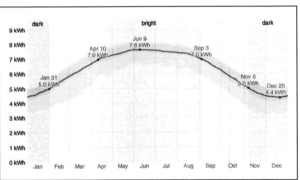

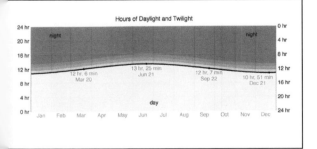

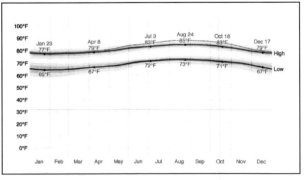

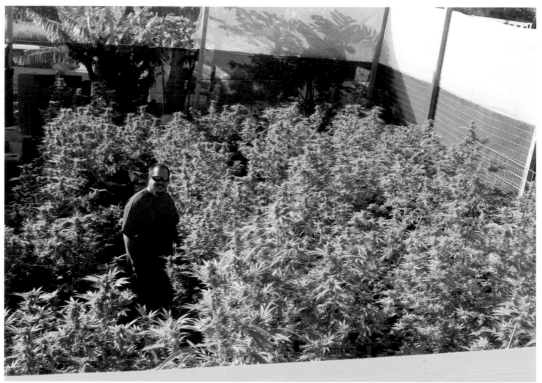

Jared in the trial Garden

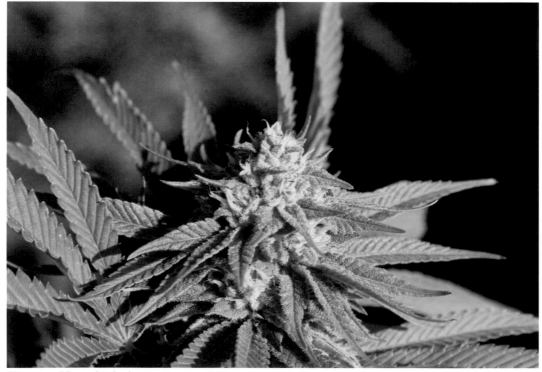

Close-up of flowering bud

plant that chemically measures the number of hours of uninterrupted darkness to determine when to begin to flower. Most varieties require 10–11 hours or less of darkness to flower. When they're placed outdoors under a natural light regimen any time in Hawaii, they begin to flower no matter the season.

I saw just two gardens while I was there. The plants were in vegetative growth, filling out a bit before they were allowed to flower. This was accomplished simply by using strategically placed fluorescent lights around the garden that were kept on all night. Once the plants grow to the desired size, the lights are turned off and the plants initiate flowering.

HOURS OF DAYLIGHT AND TWILIGHT

The minimum dark time on the first day of summer is 10 hours and 35 minutes. This is a long-enough period to force most varieties, except perhaps some equatorials, into flowering. On December 21, the shortest day, the plants are in darkness about 13 hours and 51 minutes, and receive a longer duration of light than in higher latitudes

INTENSITY OF LIGHT

The most intense light falls on Molokai on June 9. The least intense occurs on December 20, when the intensity is only 57% of the June 9 radiation.

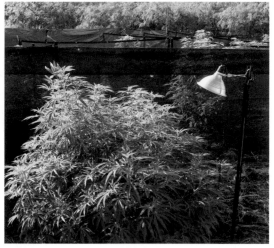

The compact fluorescent lights (CFL) were kept on all night to prevent flowering so plants could get to a larger size.

CLOUD COVER

Most of the year, with the exception of October and November, the skies are 70–80% clear to partly cloudy.

MOLOKAI TEMPERATURES THROUGHOUT THE YEAR

MONTH HIGH / LOW(°F)	RAIN
January 76° / 62°	8 days
February 76° / 62°	7 days
March 77° / 63°	6 days
April 78° / 64°	5 days
May 80° / 66°	3 days
June 81° / 68°	2 days
July 83° / 69°	3 days
August 83° / 70°	3 days
September 84° / 69°	3 days
October 82° / 68°	5 days
November 80° / 66°	6 days
December 77° / 64°	8 days

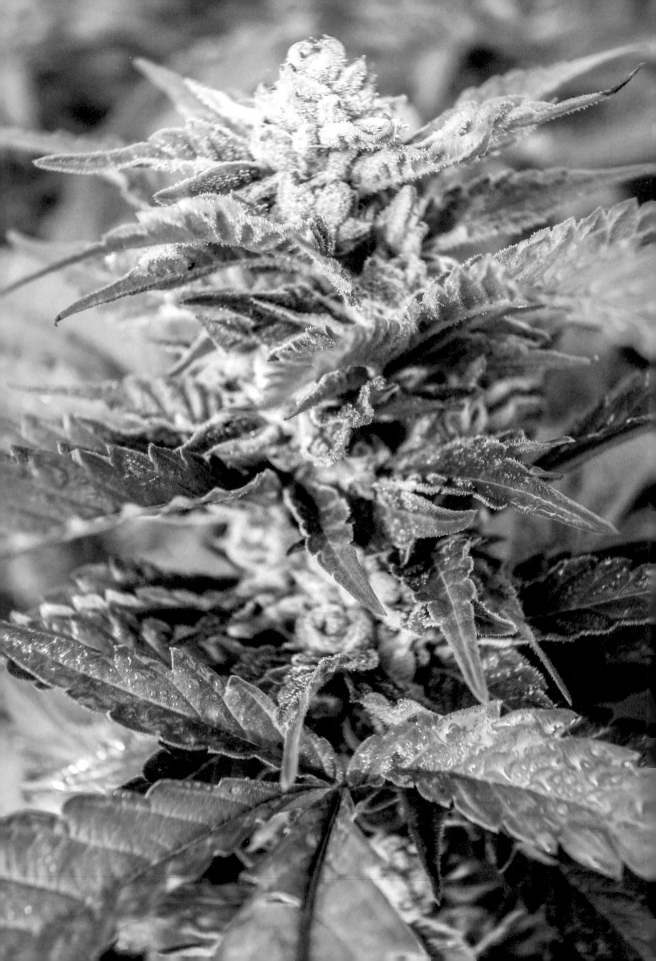

When the plants had grown fairly large, the lights were turned off. With long hours of darkness, they immediately started to flower. I was in the garden around December 4, 2017, when the plants were at the start of the flowering cycle; the lights had been turned off the previous week. I thought that it would take two months for the plants to ripen and that I would return in time for the harvest.

I should have known that that was not to be. I had forgotten that the plants were getting a far shorter light period. Longer nights speed up ripening, so the plants sacrifice bud size for shorter ripening time.

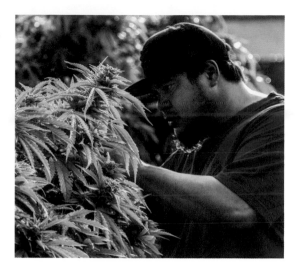

PHOTOS FROM THE HAWAIIAN GROW

My friend Zach was kind enough to take the photos you see here. They were taken on December 6, shortly before and during harvesting.

They were mostly Molokai G13; G13, a heavy, almost couch-potato indica, has a high content of pinene, which makes it sedating and relaxing. The Molokai version is lightly sprinkled with sativa genetics. This gives it a bit more energetics and more conducive to daytime, as well as evening, use.

Although people think of it as an indica, it has a mostly sativa morphology. It's a vigorous grower with a lot of spreading lateral branches, and it can easily grow 8–10 feet tall. Those characteristics indicate its substantial sativa heritage, but its effects come from its indica side.

Another sativa characteristic is continued vegetative growth during the first half of flowering. The plants fill out with continued stem growth, adding several feet and extending branching. At maturity, these plants were 8–9 feet tall and 8–10 feet wide.

G13 has a "mysterious" history. One story is that it was bred at the University of Mississippi and smuggled out. From my knowledge of the university's lab, I don't think that's a credible story. Another is that it was developed in Washington State in a federally subsidized laboratory. This rumor is persistent, but vague. The problem with that theory is that there were no labs licensed to grow in the Northwest at the time the variety broke out.

Opposite: A mature bud. Winter crop buds are on the small side because they mature quickly and don't have time for more growth.

Chapter 4

Hawaiian Legal

Covers:
- Indoors: Extending the light period for vegetating

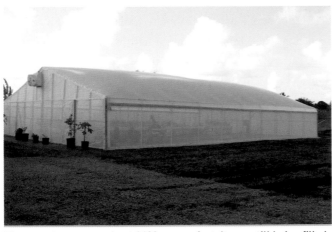

The greenhouse was about 2400 square feet. It was still being filled with plants when I visited.

I met Jason at a marijuana and health conference in Oahu. He invited me to visit his medical farm on the North Shore of Oahu. It serves about one hundred patients. With each patient allowed ten plants, Jason's Care Facility grows about one thousand plants. It's all done in a 40′ × 60′ structure, a total of 2,400 square feet. It has metal and wood framing, and is clad in 6-millimeter double polyethylene. The side walls are 10 feet high, and the peak reaches 17 feet.

The main purpose of the greenhouse is to protect plants from rain and wind. The temperature range here on Oahu is considered mild; the major problems are rain and moisture. The lowest temperatures occur in January, when the thermometer dips into the high 60s, but most of the time it ranges between the 70s and low 80s, and the temperature is no higher than the high 80s during June, July, and August.

To prevent the "greenhouse effect," when heat generated by sunlight heats up a closed area, the sides of the greenhouse are lifted during the day for airflow. They're closed at night and on rainy and windy days.

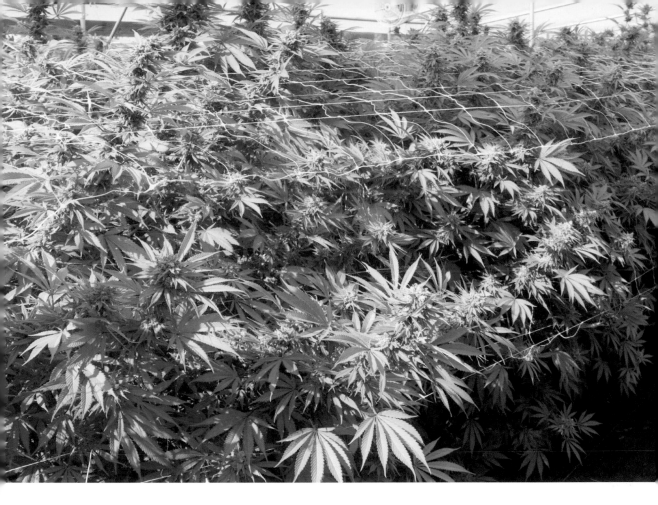

Oahu is at the 21st latitude, and there's only slight variation between summer and winter day length. On June 22, the longest day, there are just under 13.5 hours of light. On the shortest day, December 21, it's just under 11 hours. As a result, almost all plants start to flower soon after germination unless the length of the light period is extended.

Lighting the plants to prevent flowering is accomplished using compact fluorescent lights hung over the plants. They're controlled using a timer that turns the lights on most of the night.

Since it's so easy to manipulate the flowering cycle, there are plants in all stages of growth, creating a continuous supply and workflow without requiring "bulges" of temporary workers.

Jason's farm manager, Brody, mentioned that the week around the full moon has a slight effect on flowering, holding the plants back a bit. I didn't think that was the case until I looked at the full moon that night. The moon, rather than being at an acute angle in the sky, is much closer to being straight overhead. It's much brighter than it is at the 37th parallel, where I usually view it.

Jason is trying out many varieties and is especially impressed with a Chem Dog x Durban Poison, Greenpoint Seed's Indiana Bubblegum x Stardog, and their house strain Blue Dream x Gogi OG. Patients request those varieties the most.

We had come to the farm late in the afternoon. Soon dusk set in, and Jason's friends came to check out the garden. It was an absolutely great place to socialize. Yes, the fluorescents were a little glaring, but the scenery set the mood.

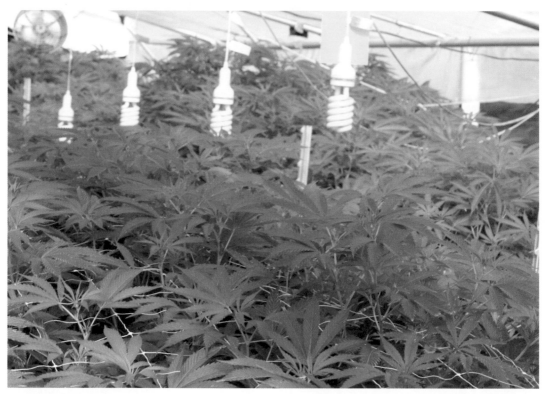

Plants in the last stage of vegetation before turning the auxiliary fluorescent lights off.

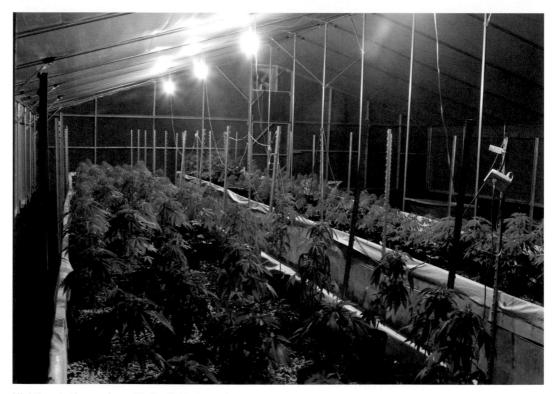

Nightime in the garden with the lights turned on.

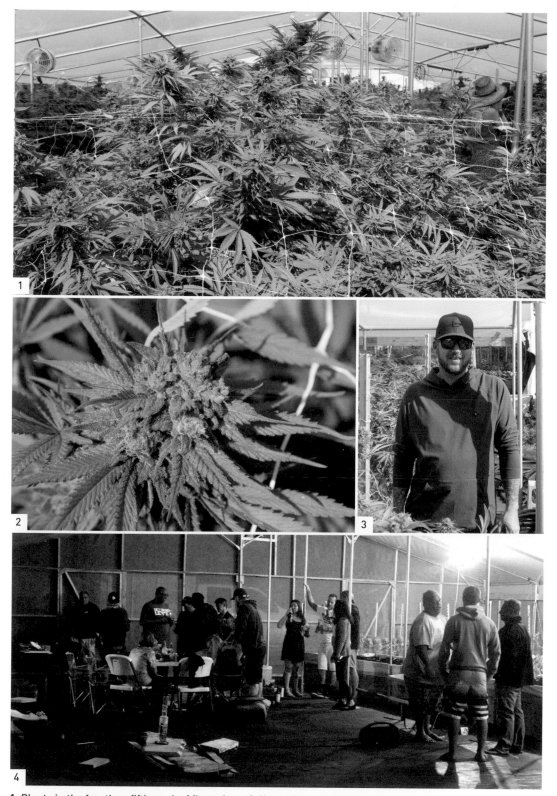

1. Plants in the fourth or fifth week of flowering.   2. Young flower almost three weeks old.
3. Jason of Hanley Care. 4. 2013 Party held for inauguration of the greenhouse. 2013 Bong city center for flower destruction.

Chapter 5

Lessons from a Jamaican Winter Garden

Covers:
- Growing in a short-day environment using close planting

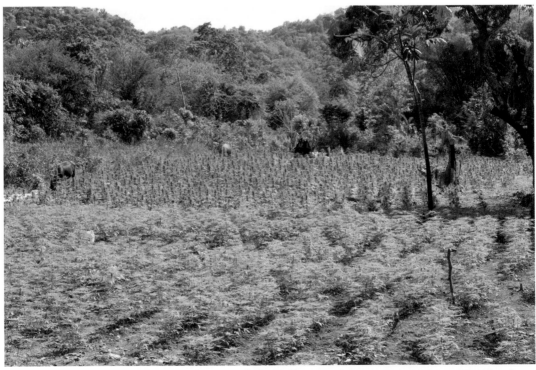

The field was about an acre. There were two sets of plants. The ones close-up were about a month old and were transitioning to flowering. For the first weeks the long night was interrupted by lighting the plants for a few moments by walking a portable light along the rows.

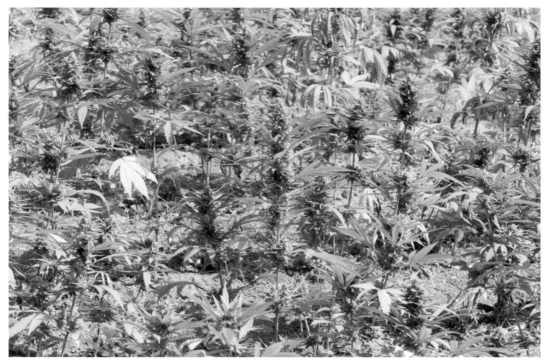

The rows were about 30" apart and the plants were spaced 3-4 inches apart in the row.

Bob Marley's dream and demand, "Legalize It!," has finally come to pass in Jamaica. People aren't going to jail for cannabis. It's used freely in more places. However, licensing legal marijuana companies is a different story. As in many states in the United States, it can be costly to go legal, so there's still a large alternative market. And naturally, the retail market is but the tip of a vertical alternative supply chain. It all starts with the farmer.

In February I took a trip to Jamaica and happened to be walking in the woods in one of the island's agricultural areas. As we made our way through brush along a rocky path, my guide casually mentioned that there was a squatter grow nearby.

I decided to make a detour and visit the pop-up farm.

The garden's perimeters were marked by barbwire that was only symbolic—it was only 4 feet high. Inside, there were rows of plants spaced about 30 inches apart, and the plants were 4–6 inches apart in the rows.

There were two groups of plants in the garden. The first group was planted from seed three to four weeks ago. The plants, all under a foot tall, were beginning to show the first signs of flowering.

The second group were plants about halfway through flowering and would be ready in three or four weeks. These plants had straight stems that ranged from 1.5 to 2.5 feet tall.

None of the plants looked particularly vigorous. The reason was that they were growing in an alkaline clay-loam soil that wasn't fertile, with nutrient insolubility and lockout caused by the clay's high pH. The field was flood irrigated, and little fertilizer, if any, was used.

Jamaica has a year-round growing season, because the weather stays warm and the sun shines most of the time. But it's close to the equator, so it has far less seasonal variation in day length than high-latitude areas. It ranges between 15 hours and 5 minutes on June 22, the first day of summer, and 9 hours and 15 minutes on December 22, the first day of winter. Most varieties respond to the long night period by changing growth from vegetative to flowering all year.

This commercial garden was not sophisticated and had lots of room for improvement. But there are things to be learned. First, early flowering and close planting both discourage plants from branching out. Instead, the plants put their energy into growing a single straight stem. When they flower, all their energy goes into growing bud along it.

Because the plant puts little time into vegetative growth, it takes less time from seed to maturity, 75–90 days. This can be duplicated outdoors using light deprivation, and indoors by limiting the vegetative period once the plants grow 10–15 inches tall, depending on variety.

Why Short Days are Relevant to You

Are you planning to grow an outdoor garden this year? Here are some ideas you can start now.

If you live in the southern tier of the country, where the temperature consistently rises to 65 degrees daily, you can plant outdoors now and year-round.

If the plants are large enough for you to consider placing them into flowering, just put them outdoors, and the long dark period (more than 10.5 hours daily) will induce them to flower. If you're gardening in the spring, toward the end of flowering the plants may need light deprivation to maintain long nights. Cover the plants to maintain the 11-hour dark period, as nights get shorter in the spring. To promote faster ripening, increase the dark period each day to 13 hours.

If you live in the northern tier and have a shorter planting season, you can plant seeds after July 1 through July 15, or clones after July 15 until mid-August. The plants will stop vegetative growth shortly after planting and grow into small plants with just a few, if any, branches, or remain a single stem. In either case, they'll be laden with buds.

Opposite: The single stems of the plants grow buds 8"-15" long. They started flowering soon after germination.

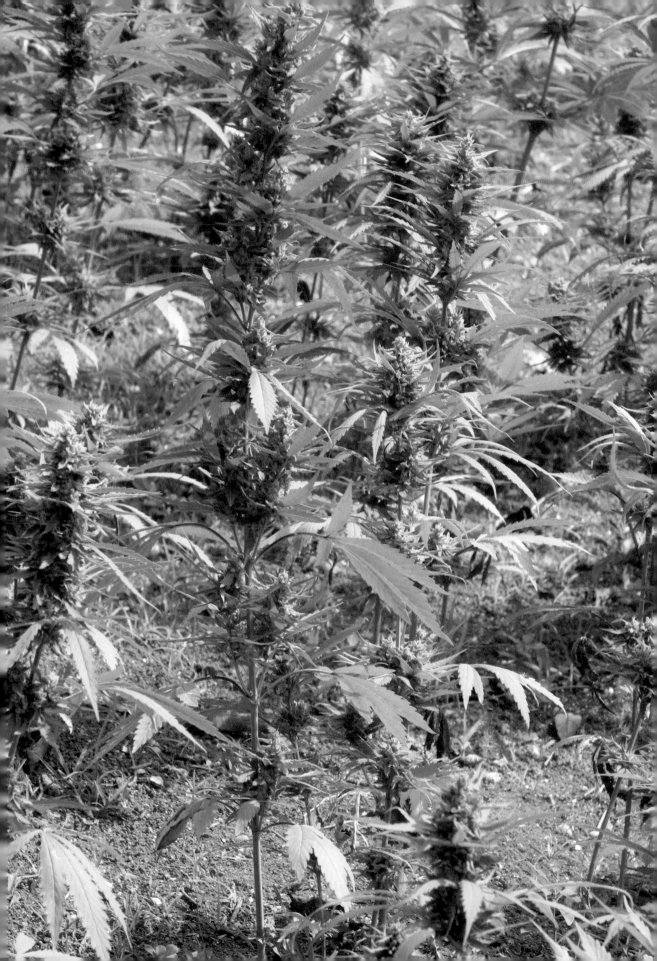

Chapter 6

Plant Regeneration: How to Achieve a Second Harvest

Regeneration—Reverting plants that have ended flowering to vegetative growth serves two uses:

1. Saving genetics- If a particular plant has genetics that you want to preserve but you haven't taken clones, reverting the plant to vegetative growth preserves the genetics.
2. It is often faster, easier, more convenient and less labor intensive than cloning or starting with seeds.

Yields from regenerated plants tend to be greater since much of their infrastructure remains intact, including the root system and part of the stem. Regenerated plants pruned of just their buds have fairly complete infrastructures, so they can be fairly sizeable without taking a lot of time in vegetative growth.

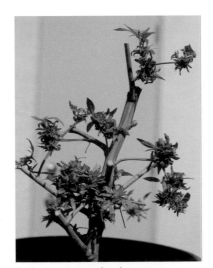

A plant regenerating from spots where vegetation had been left.

When a plant is pruned, new leaves and branches usually begin to grow within a few weeks. Marijuana gardeners can do the same thing with their plants. The regeneration process begins at harvest. There is no seed sowing or repotting involved. When harvesting, take the buds but leave at least a few branches with some leaf material and immature buds on them. The more you leave, the larger the plant will be when it starts growing again. The rest of the

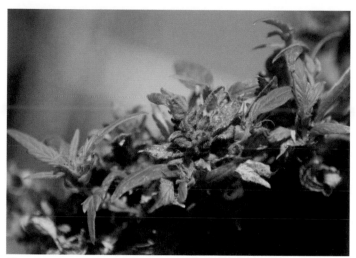

Close-up of first vegetative growth after the lighting cycle had been changed to vegetative. The light was on constantly.

plant can be harvested as usual.

It is important that vegetative material is left on the branches because the plant won't regenerate without it.

Gardeners who wish to grow single-stem plants should remove all but one branch or leaf site on the stem and remove the others. The plants' energy will focus on this remaining growth site.

Once the plants are harvested, the lights should be left on continuously. The plants will switch to the vegetative cycle and start to grow again in about 10 days. Then they can be kept in the vegetative regimen of continuous light to serve as clone mothers or they can be forced to flower when they reach the desired size.

Regenerated plants tend to sprout many branches, which results in a bushy plant with many small buds. To grow larger buds, prune the plants so that there are fewer branches. The plant will put its energy into the remaining branches, resulting in fewer, but bigger buds.

Most people practice regeneration only once or twice and then start again with new plants. One popular method is to harvest an indoor plant and then place it outdoors in the spring or summer. The

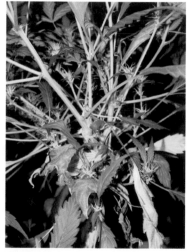

First new growth on this plant was still flowering.

plant regenerates and produces a fall harvest. In warmer climates you can place plants outdoors for a winter or spring harvest and then let them regenerate for fall harvest. If plants are forced to flower in spring or early summer using light deprivation, they can be pruned for regeneration and they will flower again in the fall.

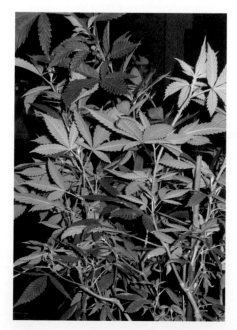

After several weeks the plant reverted to full vegetative growth.

Chapter 7

Tweaking Bud Potency Using UV Light

This room is illuminated using tanning lamps. Usually they are used 5 hours a day in conjunction with HPS lamps. In this photo the HPS lamps have been turned off for illustrative purposes.

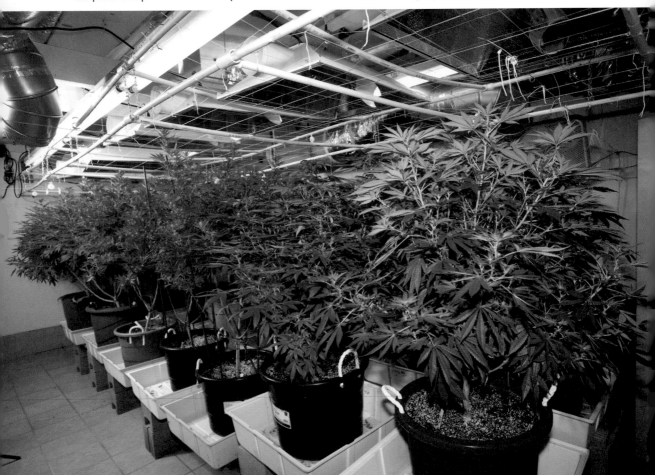

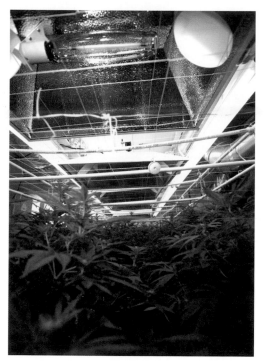

A view of the room showing the 6 foot tanning lamps.

HOW PLANTS UTILIZE LIGHT

People used to think that plants were vegetables: that they have no way of reacting quickly to their environment and were more like couch potatoes with very slow reactions. There were always clear signs that this isn't necessarily so. Sunflowers track so their flowers always face the sun. The Venus fly-trap closes on its victims the moment it's touched. Mimosa pudica, the sensitive plant, collapses its leaves after being touched. But when it's touched repeatedly by the same stimulus, it becomes habit-uated and stops reacting. After not stimulating the plant for weeks, it still "remembered" the stimulus and didn't react. It had "learned." Most important to us, a fraction of a second after lights are turned on, plants start photosynthesizing.

Rhodopsin is a pigment sensitive to light. A version is found in bacteria, and it's used in the so-phisticated human visual system. It's also found in plants and helps cannabis to regulate its flowering by distinguishing light from dark periods.

Plants also share stress responses with animals regarding UV light. Dark skin has high melanin content to protect against UV light. Light-skinned people develop more intense stress reactions and respond to the light by producing melanin, causing tanning or, more severely, sunburn, which actu-ally results in the destruction of layers of skin and other damaging reactions.

Plants growing under natural sunlight develop resistance to these harmful UV rays in several ways. They grow longer protective cells (palisade cells) to disperse the light to mini-mize its intensity, and they produce higher levels of pigments, flavonoids, and terpenes as sun shields. In various experiments and anecdotal reports, THC production increased by 10%. Terpene levels also increase signifi-cantly. There are positive effects in

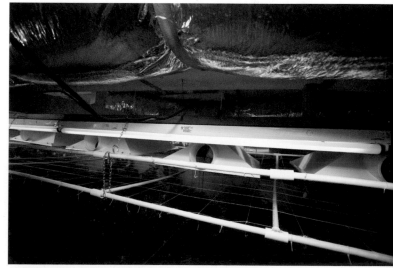

A tanning lamp with reflector.

other plants, too. For instance, tomatoes grow thicker skins and contain more solids and flavonoids.

When plants grown indoors are placed outdoors in late spring or summer, they sometimes get sunburned. Their leaves droop or dry out, and they suffer tissue damage. Whether or not they survive and thrive, it's a setback. For this reason, plants should be gently, gradually introduced to direct sun, perhaps first by placing them in the shade or by using shade cloth to protect against the sun's intensity.

You might think that plants in greenhouses are getting full sun. However, most plastics and glass are opaque to UV light. One exception is acrylic sheet, often known by its brand-name Plexiglas.

Indoors, fluorescents, and HPS lamps produce no UV light. Metal halide lamps often produce small but significant amounts of UV, but the plate glass required for safely enclosing the lamp in the reflector is opaque to it.

Some LED manufacturers include the spectrum in their mixes, but emitters in these spectrums are still costly.

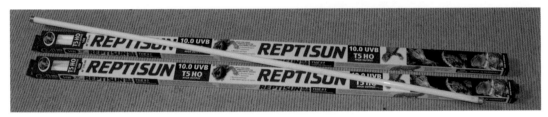

Reptile lights can be used to supply UV light.

What's a person to do?
- A handy friend decided to use tanning lamps that advertised deep bronzing. All the parts were available, but he had to construct the holders and wire the ballasts to the lamp holders. He used the equivalent of one tube for each 1000-watt HPS.
- Fluorescent reptile lamps rated 10X emit UV light that the plants require. These lamps can be used on a one-to-one basis.
- UV lamps geared specifically for horticulture are available online.

The lamps need only be used during the last twenty to thirty days of flowering, for 6 hours a day. For instance, plants growing outdoors receive the highest amount of UV light in the summer, when they're in the vegetative stage. I haven't seen the results of any experimentation on this. This is an area where there's a lot of room for trials.

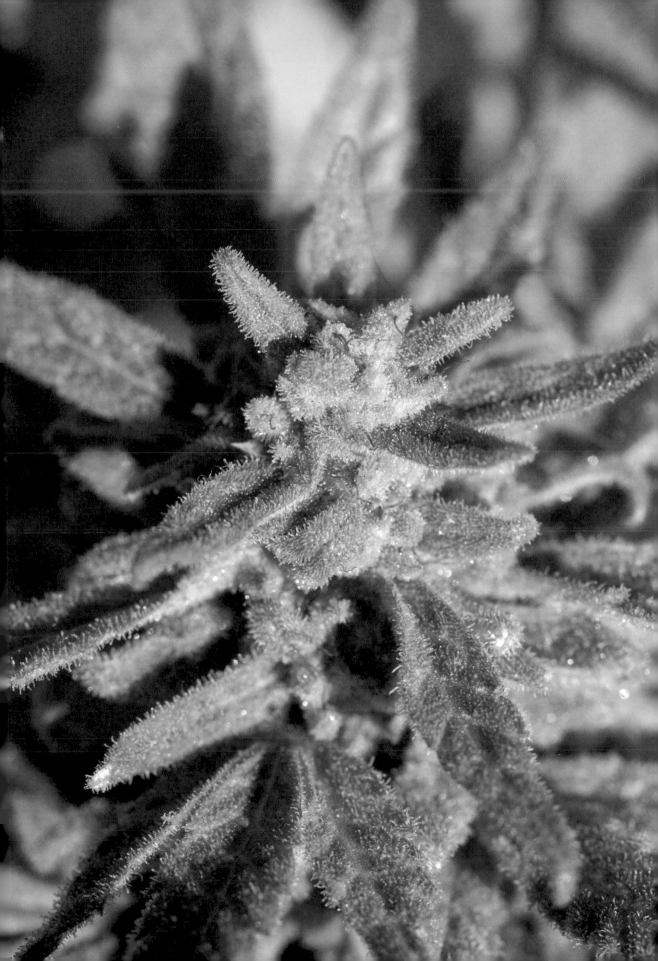

Chapter 8

Summer Interlude: Wick System in my Greenhouse

Covers:
- The low-water, easy-to-care-for wick system
- Manicuring and drying

GETTING NEW PLANTS

It was the end of June, and the 4' × 8' space in the greenhouse was empty. A friend of mine had some extra Purple Pineapple plants that he passed on to me. This variety has a unique quality: when it gets more than 4 hours of darkness, it initiates flowering.

I collected the plants near the end of June. They were in 6-inch containers. I added nylon wicks to the bottom of each container to make them self-watering by drawing water from the reservoir below. The twenty-five plants were about 15 inches high. They were growing outdoors during the day to get the sun's free rays and then before sundown were placed in an indoor space illuminated by HPS lamps. Thus they received light constantly.

As soon as I placed them in the greenhouse, June 22, the longest day of the year, the plants started to flower because they were receiving only about 15 hours of light and 9 hours of darkness. No light deprivation was needed. To keep them from flowering, I would have had to interrupt the dark cycle with light every hour. This variety will start to flower if it gets more than 4 hours of unin-

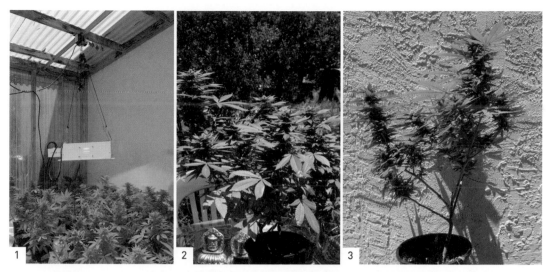

1. The plants in the greenhouse get supplemental light during the day.   2. Before trimming. 3. After trimming the plants were pruned of extraneous vegetation to center their energy on growing buds.

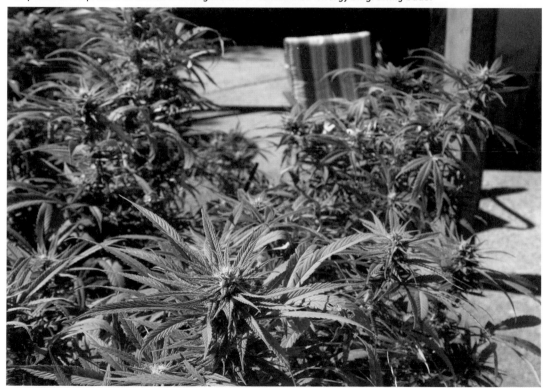

Plants in early flowering in greenhouse.

terrupted darkness. I used a repeating timer with a 4-foot fluorescent light to turn on for 1 minute every hour.

The additional light was a 1000-watt HPS lamp on a light mover that was placed about 15 inches over the canopy. It supplements the natural light when the greenhouse is in shade, from 8 a.m. to 12 noon and then from 3 to 6 p.m. This helped the plants develop bigger, more potent buds.

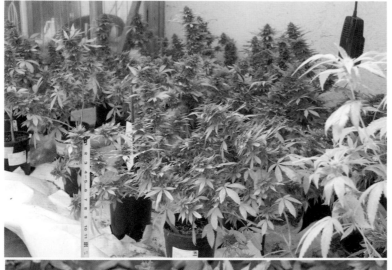

The garden is ready to harvest. All the plants were clones so they all matured at the same time.

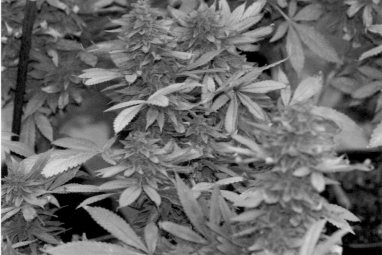

All the buds on the plants had received light so they were all mature.

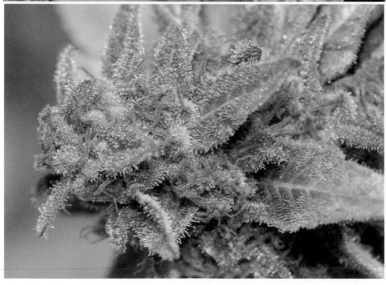

Close-up of a bud.

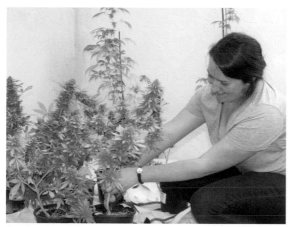

Cutting the plants was an easy task. A pruner was used.

MY UNIQUE HYDRO GARDEN SETUP

The plants were self-watered using nylon wicks to draw water up from a reservoir underneath to the planting mix. So flushing was a simple task. The tap water here originates as runoff, rather than from a well, so it has a mineral content of only about 70 ppm, which is very low. Twice during the week before harvest I ran tap water through the 6-inch containers until about 20% of it drained out. As it soaked through the containers, soluble salts dissolved in the water and drained away, so the roots had a chance to sip clear water. This didn't remove nutrients from the plants, but they used up what was in their systems.

HARVEST DAY

August 28 was harvest day. Twenty-five of the twenty-eight Purple Pineapple (PP) plants were cut. The other three plants were reserved for other experiments or photography. There were three very obvious signs that the plants were ripe.

Now the time had come. The buds were ripe: HARVEST!

Postscript: The water in the reservoir, which contains the extra nutrients from the double flush, has been pumped into a holding container. I dilute it a bit and use it to feed my garden plants.

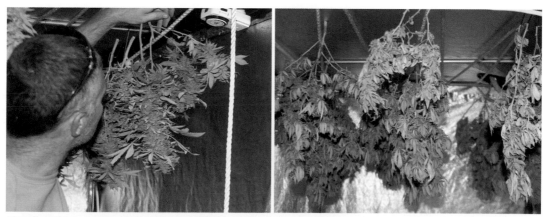

The plants were hung to dry and cure over five or six weeks. Then they will be manicured. The room stays in the 60's to low 70's, with moderate humidity.

Chapter 9

Building Wick Systems

An Easy Way to Grow

Covers:
- The most environmentally friendly setup

The wick container system is an easy way to garden because it's self-watering and removes the uncertainty of when to water. It requires far less care than hand watering, and it's simple, fast to assemble, and inexpensive to set up.

The wick system is based on capillary action. One example of this is a tissue drawing up water from a puddle. The system we set up works on the same principle. Instead of tissue, we use braided nylon rope.

EQUIPMENT NEEDED TO BUILD A WICK SYSTEM

Starting from the bottom, we need a tray that's at least 3 inches deep and wide enough to support the plant container. The wider the container, the deeper the tray should be. For instance, with a 6-foot container, I use a 10-inch-deep tray, but with small containers the tray is only 3–5 inches deep.

Next, we need some blocks to hold the container a few inches above the tray. Some possibilities are 2′ × 4′ or 4′ × 4′ boards, Styrofoam blocks, or an inverted plastic tray.

The container is next. Select the same size container that you would normally use. I've used

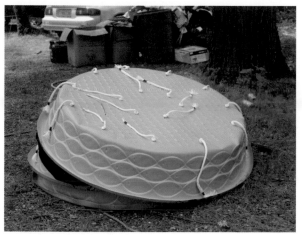

Holes were drilled in the tray for the wicks.

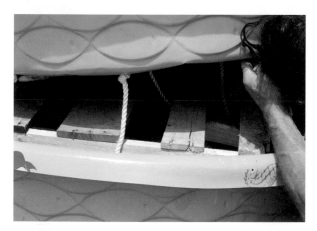

Pallets were used to support tray above the water. followed by

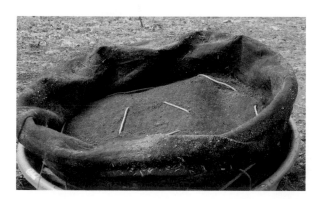

this system with 4-inch containers and 8-foot-wide soft containers.

Next is the wick. Nylon braided rope draws up water very well. These wicks last for a long time. I've used some more than 10 years. Select the wick size. The larger the container, the thicker the wick should be. A small container needs only a ¼-inch wick, while a large container, which is deeper than the small, can use wicks up to ¾ inches. Wider containers should have more wicks, so water is drawn across the entire bottom of the container by the wicks.

Next, the planting mix goes into the container. Once the water is drawn up the wick to the bottom of the soil level, the soil starts wicking it up vertically 8–10 inches. Many mixes are able to draw the moisture up, so try your favorite first. You probably have already seen the soil mix wicking when you watered a plant and excess water dripped into the tray below. A while later, the water disappeared as it was pulled up into the planting mix. The wick system works in the same way.

INSTALLATION

- Place the wood or plastic supports in the tray.
- Measure and cut the wick. It should start at the bottom of the tray, go through the drain hole in the container and stretch across the container bottom to the drainage hole on the other side and down to the bottom of the tray. The rope tends to fray at the ends. To prevent this, before you cut, use two twist ties, one for each end of the rope, to hold

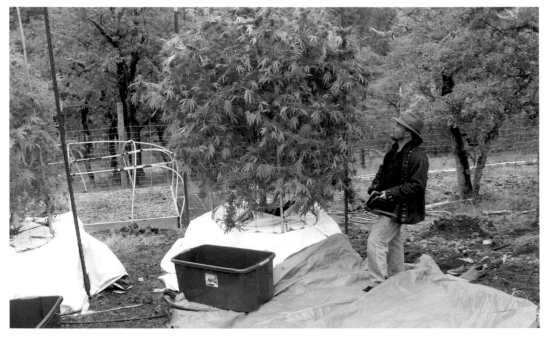

The wick system can support large plants.

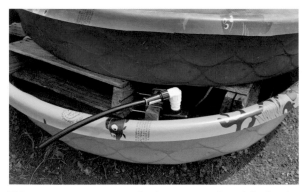

This system was automated using a reservoir and flush valve.

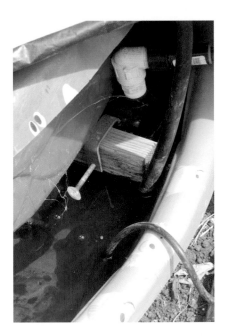

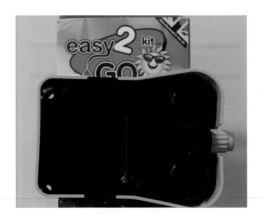

This small valve regulates water level in the reservoir.

it in place.

- If the container is wide, use two wicks, one in each set of two opposite holes. You may have to drill holes in wider containers, such as kiddie pools or wide trays. Figure that each wick drop covers about 2 square feet.
- Fill the container with planting mix.
- Plant the plant or seeds.

MAINTENANCE

- To start, add water to the container until it starts to drip into the tray.
- Fill the tray with water.
- Refill the tray as it loses water. You can also water the container from the top once in a while.
- The planting mix absorbs water from the wick automatically as the plant uses it.

OPTIONS

This system can be automated. By placing a reservoir above the container level and placing a flush valve in the tray, the water level can be maintained for a longer time.

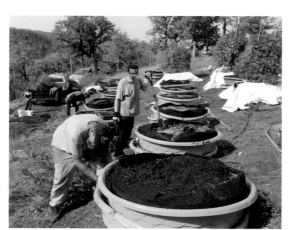

A number of trays can be connected to a reservoir so the whole garden is irrigated just by filling the reservoir. The advantage to this system is that each tray receives water only as it needs it.

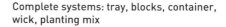

Complete systems: tray, blocks, container, wick, planting mix

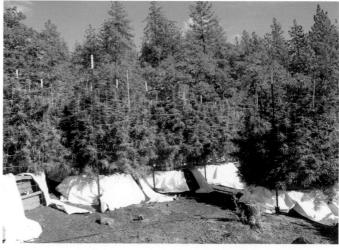

Chapter 10

The Benefits of Small Plants

A large, healthy, flowering marijuana plant is an inspiring sight. It's the successful culmination of a season's effort. The quest for big plants is an artifact of eased prohibition rules, which allowed cultivation for personal use, usually based on four, six, or ten plants allowed. Some of these numbers have remained with legalization. If you can grow only a limited number of plants, grow as big as you can. However, commercial growers, even microbusinesses, can sometimes grow an unlimited number of plants. This opens up a lot of possibilities.

Growing a large plant takes time, labor, energy, and space. The first stages of growth are spent growing infrastructure, that is, branches and leaves. These parts of the plant are not harvested. Only the flowers grown on the branches during flowering are used.

When figuring the cost of the active ingredient, whether THC or another cannabinoid, all the costs must be taken into account. This includes the cost of getting the plants ready for flowering.

There's a way to speed up production and save time, energy, and labor: remove growing plant infrastructure from the equation so the plants spend more time flowering.

Usually, vegetating plants grow until the canopy space is filled. These plants will keep growing vegetatively as long as they're provided light, 18–24 hours daily. Assuming you have set up that light, fill the canopy with plants placed close together, on 6–8-inch centers. Once they're in place, grow them vegetatively until they have 5–8 sets of leaves. Use a timer to change the light cycle to 12 hours on, 12 hours off. Make sure not to interrupt the dark period with any light other than green because it will interrupt the plants' photoperiod regimen, resulting in softer, smaller buds.

The plants will start flowering within 7–10 days. Some varieties with sativa backgrounds will continue to grow for a while even as they flower, doubling in height by ripening time. Other varieties, mostly with indica backgrounds, slow vertical growth almost immediately, growing about 20% taller.

The plantlets of most varieties will not grow any side branches once they're in flowering regimen. Instead, they'll put their energy into producing flowers along the stem that ripen into a single or just a few large buds.

This technique can be used indoors or out. Indoors under lights, it's easy to adjust the light regimen. Outdoors and in greenhouses, use a blackout curtain for light deprivation during the summer. During the fall, winter, and early spring there's a long-enough dark period to promote flowering.

With small plants you save transplanting, pruning, staking, and other laborious chores; cut greenhouse shelf time; and save on manicuring because there are fewer buds that are larger and easier to manicure.

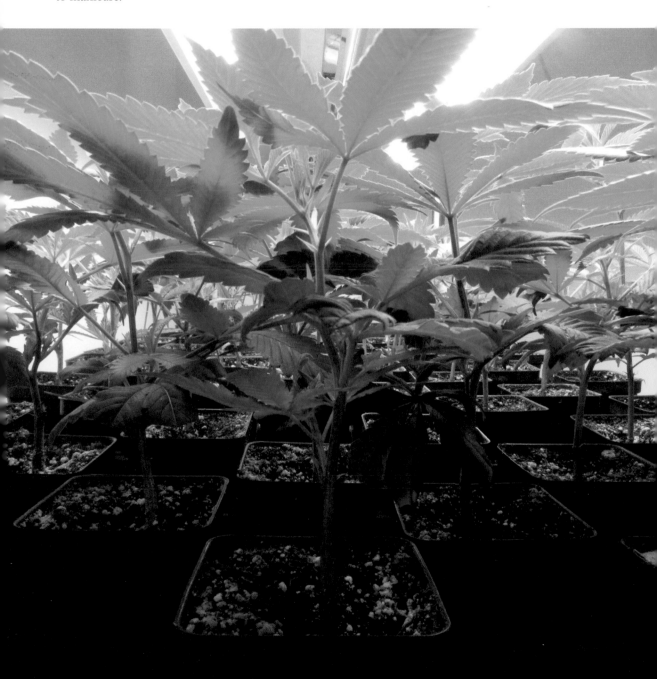

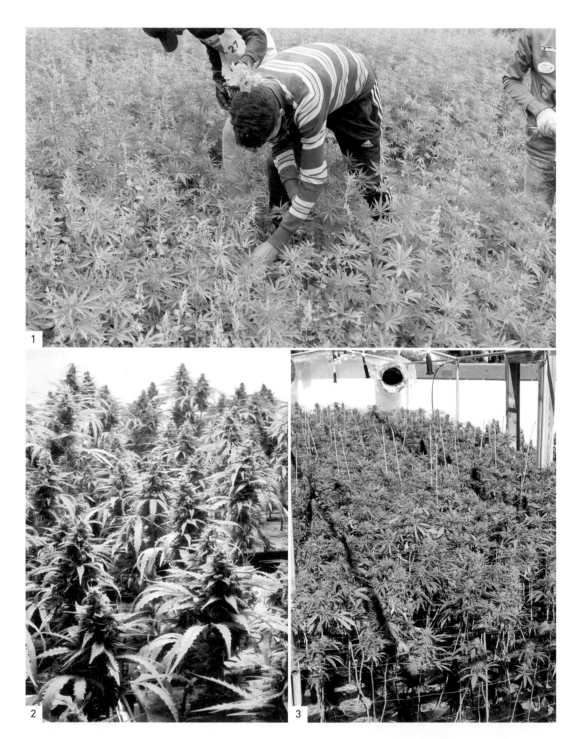

1. In Jamaica males are removed from the field to feed the goats. In mid-July the male plants' flowers were opening and the females were 2 weeks into flowering. The seeds had been broadcast and there were 10-15 plants per square foot. By harvest time the males will be desiccated, leaving half that number of plants to be harvested.   2. Indica dominant hybrid clones were set in 4" rockwool cubes and placed under an HID light using a 12/12 light/dark regimen. Each produced a single big bud.   3. Single-stemmed plants, tightly planted.

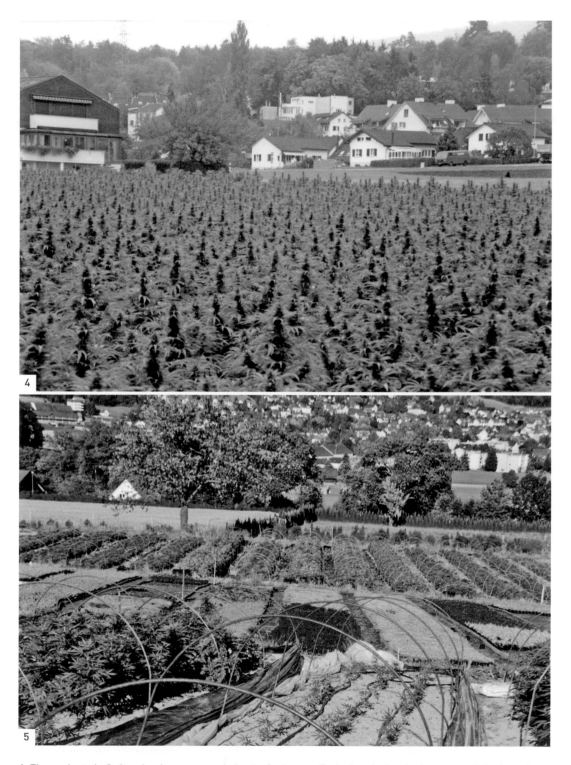

4. These plants in Switzerland were spaced about a foot apart. Each plant had a single stem and single main bud.   **5.** A Swiss field showing different sections of the garden

Chapter 11

Cannabis Seeds or Clones:
Which is Right for You?

THERE ARE TWO WAYS TO START A CANNABIS GARDEN— USING EITHER SEEDS OR CLONES

For most gardeners, it is faster and easier to work with clones than seeds. Just think of your home garden. You are much more likely to start with young plants rather than seeds. They are faster and easier to start than it is to germinate seeds. Also, plants of the same variety from seeds can vary in quality, but clones have already been selected and are uniform.

In many states where marijuana is legal or is allowed medical dispensaries sell clones. In Northern California at least, the clone companies produce infection and disease-free clones. If you have access to healthy clones start with them.

If you don't have access to clones locally, look online where you will find many clone and seed sources that will ship to you. They provide a much wider choice of varieties including fabled strains not available locally. Although ordering seeds is not totally risk-free, the small package is unlikely to be detected because seeds have no odor and are shipped in "normal" envelopes that don't raise suspicions.

ADVANTAGES OF SEEDS

- Plants from seeds grow a better tap-root than clones. The taproot is the equivalent of the main stem. It grows straight down with lateral branches growing along its length. A deep tap-root reaches the water table or moist soil at a lower level of topsoil or penetrable subsoil.

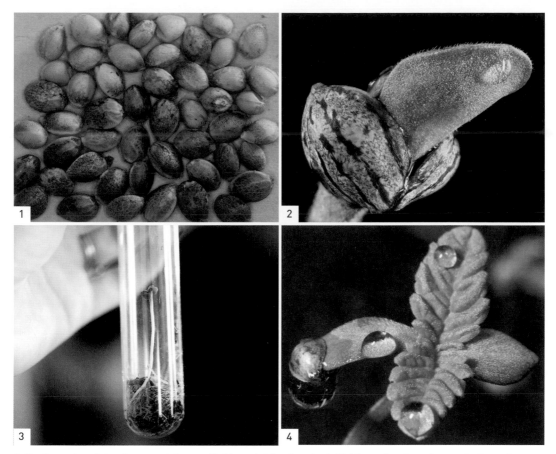

1. Each seed contains the complete genetic blueprint for the plant. Lighter colored seeds may be immature. Darker colored seeds are mature. [Photo: Lizzy Cozzi] **2.** Seed germinating. Its first leaves, called cotyledons, emerge. [Photo: Professor P] **3.** Seedling germinating in a test tube. [Photo: Lizzy Cozzi] **4.** The first set of true leaves grows within a few days. [Photo: Professor P]

- Seeds are free from disease and pests, including viruses. Clones can transfer both pests and disease.
- You know you have the variety you wanted when it comes from the seed company.
- Seeds are the product of sexual reproduction so they inherit genetic characteristics from both parents. Plants from seed exhibit some genetic variation, so you can choose the best plant or the one you like the most. Growing from seed is more adventurous, because you are not sure exactly how the plants will turn out.
- Seeds of many varieties are readily available in shops, dispensaries, by mail and over the internet. When they come from a seed company, you can have confidence in getting a variety with the basic characteristics you want.
- They are very portable and easy to store for long periods of time.

DISADVANTAGES OF SEEDS

- Marijuana has separate male and female plants. Unless they are used for breeding, males are of no use and are dangerous pollinators that endanger the potency of the female flowers with the risk of pollination.

- Usually about half the plants are males that have to be detected and removed. This can be an arduous task and the consequence of missing one can be seedy buds throughout the garden.

FEMINIZED SEEDS

Feminized seeds have been bred to produce only female plants. They are the solution to the problem of sexing males since all the plants are females.

Germinating seeds is a more delicate operation than transplanting clones.

Seeds take longer to grow and be ready to flower because rooted clones are already biologically mature and have a head start on root development.

Plants from seeds don't reproduce exactly their parents' traits. Seeds from a variety you saw and tasted will not grow to be exactly the same as their mother, though it will be a close approximation.

Because you will discard roughly half of the plants once they can be sexed, growing from seeds can more easily put you over any legal plant count limits, or leave you with fewer plants than allowed or anticipated.

ADVANTAGES OF CLONES

- Clones are taken from female plants so they are female, too. There are no males or hermaphrodites to mess with the buds.
- Clones get you past the germination "hump" that seeds present. Seeds take several weeks to catch up to a rooted rooted to replace plants as they are placed into flowering.

DISADVANTAGES OF CLONES

- Clones are only available commercially in some states that have medical marijuana laws.
- Clones of the particular variety that you would like are not always available, even where they are legal.

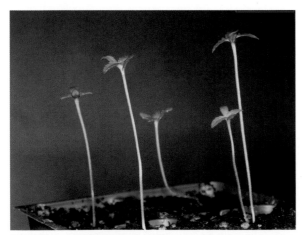
Stretching seedlings aren't getting enough light. The stems will strengthen when the plants are exposed to brighter light and air circulation.

- Clones can carry diseases and pests that can infect your whole garden. Clones from friends are more likely to be infected than professionally grown clones.

DISADVANTAGES FOR OUT-DOOR GROWER

- Clones do not grow as vigorously as seed grown plants, especially outdoors, because clones do not grow a taproot. They only grow secondary roots from the stem and subsequently most of their growth is lat-

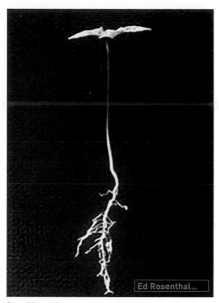

Seedlings have a strong taproot and a straight line to move liquids up and down.

eral rather than downward. The main advantage of having a taproot is the ability to dig deep into the ground and reach water not available closer to the surface. The taproot grows lateral branches along its entire length providing the plant with a network of roots that occupies a larger three-dimensional area. The result is that there are more roots in several layers of soil so they can obtain more water and nutrients to support the plant's growth. This doesn't affect plants grown inside as much because the plants don't grow as large and the taproot isn't as important in a container environment.

• The taproot on plants grown from seed is an extension of the stem so it anchors the plant and holds the canopy securely. Clone plants have a single layer of lateral roots. The stem ends close to the soil line, where it was cut. This doesn't provide as much support as a plant with a taproot.

• Outdoors, or indoors with older plants, one or two lateral roots may become dominant and develop into short tap roots that help to anchor the plant and also produce lateral roots. Their connection to the stem is reinforced from layers of growth.

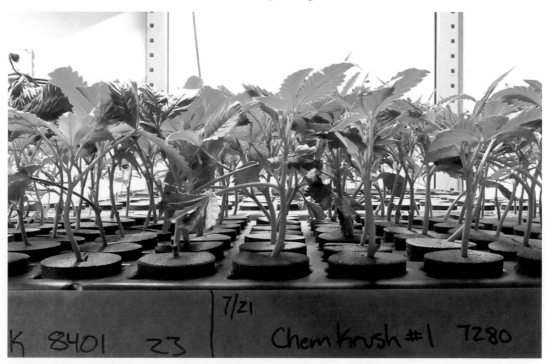

A tray of clones. The plants all have the same genetics and will grow nearly identically.

Chapter 12

Your Essential Guide to When Cannabis Buds Are Ready to Harvest

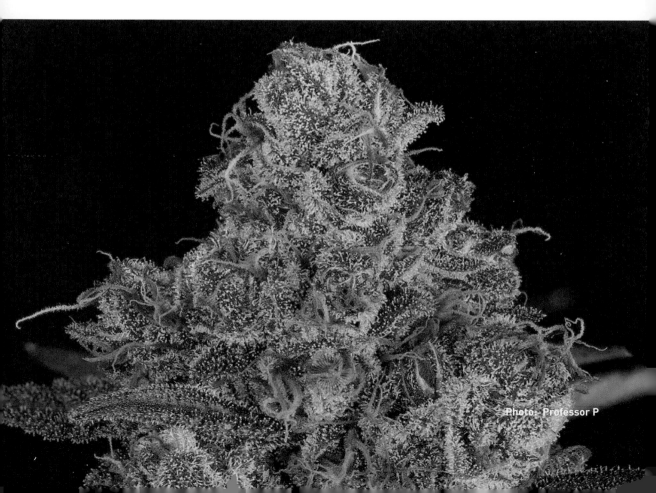

Photo: Professor P

NO BUD SHOULD BE PICKED BEFORE ITS TIME

Plants and varieties differ in maturation patterns.

Some mature all at once, so that the whole plant can be picked. Other varieties mature from the top down, or alternately, from the outside in. For these varieties, the buds on the outside mature faster than inner buds hidden from the light. Once the outer buds are harvested, the inner branches are exposed to light and quickly ripen. It can take two weeks of choosing mature buds before the plant is totally picked. Picking the plant a little at a time ensures that every bud is at maximum potency and quality.

A plant's flowering cycle, and its ripening and harvesting-time, are variety specific. Each variety is programmed to respond to a critical period of darkness that turns growth from vegetative to flowering.

Indoors, this is accomplished when the lights are cut back to twelve hours. Outdoors, the critical time period varies between about nine and eleven hours of darkness.

In addition to genetics, flowering time is also affected by light intensity and total light received on a daily basis, ambient temperature and nutrients.

Cannabis Bud Ripening Facts

- Plants of the same variety flower and ripen at about the same time. Clones from a single plant grown under the same conditions flower and ripen at the same time.
- Flowering time is determined by the light regimen, not a plant's age or size.
- When all the buds on small plants get direct sun, they tend to ripen at the same time.
- Buds on large plants that are directly lit, whether on the top of the plant or the sides, mostly ripen at the same time.
- Outdoors, big plants grown with large spaces between them will often get light from three different sides as the sun moves around them, specifically from the east, west and south. This light pattern is especially prevalent in the fall when the sun is at an acute angle and lower on the horizon.
- On large colas, outer buds often ripen while the inner buds are deprived of direct sunlight.

WHAT IS THE BEST WAY TO DETERMINE YOUR CANNABIS PICKING TIME?

Watch the development of the trichomes. Trichomes are the stalk-like resin glands that contain the active compounds, which grow on the leaves surrounding the flowers.

The flower area becomes covered with resin glands over time.

The length of this stage of growth usually lasts two to three weeks; in modern varieties these glands ripen in seven to nine weeks from flower initiation.

Late-season and long-maturing varieties usually spend about three to five weeks in this period of heavy trichome growth.

As flowers near ripeness, their caps swell with resin and the trichomes become more prominent and stand erect.

The viscous, sticky liquid that accumulates contains terpenes and cannabinoids, which are produced on the inside membrane of the trichome cap. As the resin accumulates in the cap, the flower odor becomes more intense.

The odor reaches its peak at the same time the trichomes begin to fluoresce in the light, twinkling like little crystals. In some varieties, the trichomes are so prominent that the whole bud sparkles. Using a magnifying glass, a photographer's loupe or a microscope, monitor the buds' progression to the peak of ripeness by watching the resin in the gland tops.

Under magnification, you can see individual glands turning from clear to amber or a cloudy white. These colors indicate that THC is beginning to degrade into two other cannabinoids, cannabicyclol (CBL) and cannabinol (CBN), which are not nearly as psychotropic as THC.

When the trichomes begin to change from clear to amber or cloudy white, the buds should be harvested—this is the peak moment.

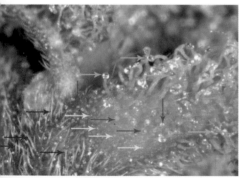

→ capitate stalked gland → capitate sessile glands
→ bulbous trichomes → cystolith hairs

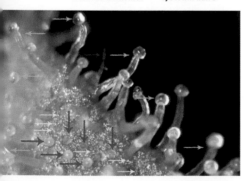

The Different Types Of Trichomes

Stalked Capitate Glandular Trichomes: These trichomes are the most abundant and contain the desired cannabinoids, terpenoids and flavonoids that growers seek.

Bulbous Trichomes: These trichomes have no stalk and are much smaller than the other trichomes. They appear mostly on leaves rather than in the bud area, especially during vegetative growth, and contain cannabinoids.

Crysolith Trichome: These trichomes do not contain cannabinoids. They grow on the bottom of the leaves to deter pests.

Sessile Stalked Capitate Trichome: These trichomes appear during the vegetative growth stage and produce only small amounts of cannabinoids.

Ripe cannabis reeks of pungent terpenes and each day brings increased intensity of odor.

Rub the leaves surrounding the bud between clean fingers and inhale. This releases aroma molecules while leaving fingers sticky with resin.

Inhale and smell an exotic medley of familiar and unusual odors that may range from sweet to acrid with outlying musks and skunks.

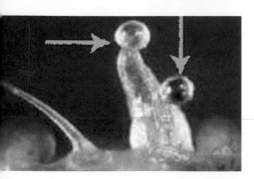

Left: Magnification of glands along surface of leaf. Red-cystolith hair; green-capitate gland heads, one of which has been decapitated.

STAGES OF FLOWERING

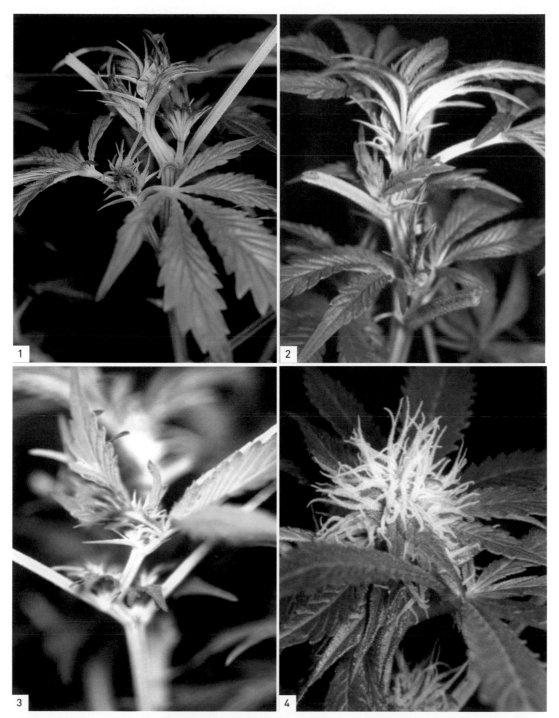

Weeks 1 & 2: The stigmas, the white or cream-colored "hairs" first appear and begin to proliferate. Stigmas are hollow tubes covered with tiny brush-like appendages. They sift the air for suitable pollen. When one attaches to a stigma, it is stripped of its sperm, which slides down the hollow tube to meet the egg.
Weeks 3 & 4: The stigmas continue to grow, forming dense clumps of "buds."

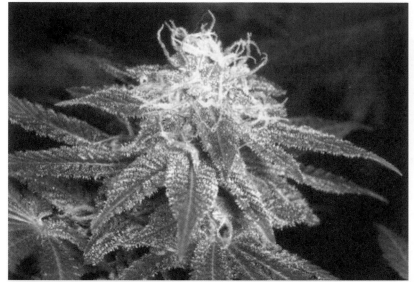

Week 6: The bud begins to ripen. While new stigmas continue to grow, older ones are drying up, turning red or tan. At the same time the stalked tricomes, which have been growing along the vegetation surrounding the stigmas, begin to stand out prominently as their caps fill with cannabinoids and terpenes manufactured along the cell membrane.

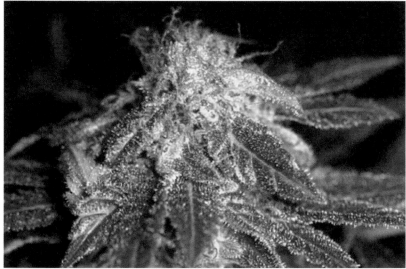

Week 7: The stigmas continue to swell with resin. The caps stretch as they fill. The plants release tricomes, that fill the area with herbal aromas.

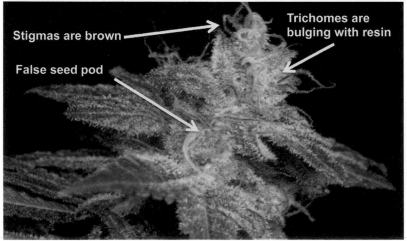

Stigmas are brown

Trichomes are bulging with resin

False seed pod

Week 8: The stigmas have all dried. The trichome caps are swelled with resin. A few have changed to a milky or amber color. The aroma is intense. Sometimes the flowers swell as if they were carrying seed. The bud is ripe.

CLOSE-UPS

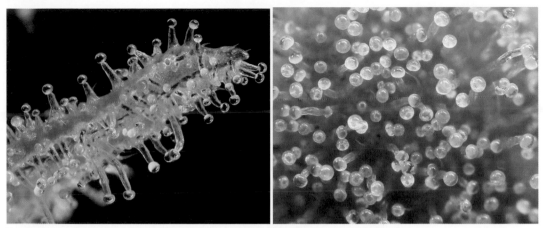

Premature - The glands are all clear and the caps are filling, but are not filled.

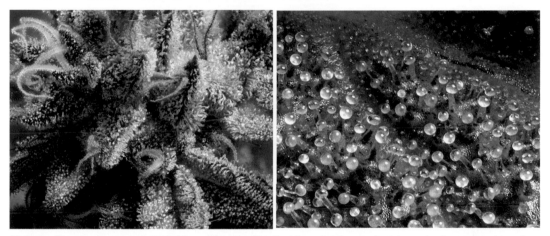

Mature - The gland caps are stretching with resin. The first few glands are changing color from clear to amber or cloudy. Time to harvest.

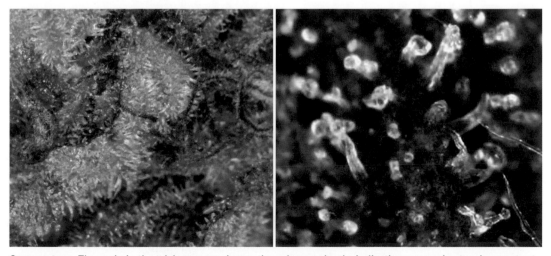

Over-mature: The resin in the trichome caps is mostly amber or cloudy, indicating conversion to a less-potent cannabinoid. The caps are breaking away from the stalks and the odor of the plant is changing to "over-ripe." Harvest immediately.

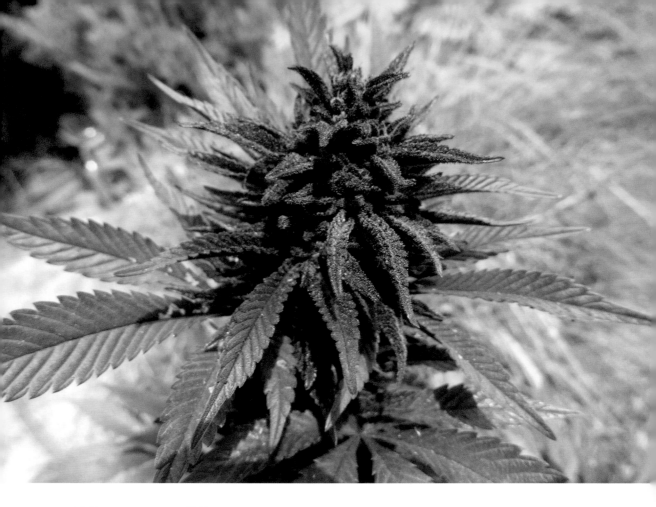

Chapter 13

California Winter Garden

Covers:
- Starting clones in a greenhouse
- How to have a successful spring harvest

SETTING UP THE GREENHOUSE

It's mid-January, and here in San Francisco's East Bay the weather is mostly cloudy with a high of 63 degrees and a low of 45. The same weather is forecast for the next five days. This doesn't sound like the most conducive weather to grow marijuana outdoors. However, during much of the mild winter

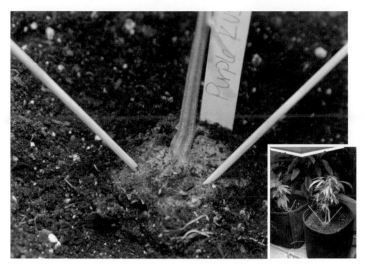

The clone cube top was positioned just above the soil line to keep the stem dry. Two skewers were used to hold the cube firmly in place. After a few days, the roots grow into the soil and the skewers are no longer needed. **2.** The light was placed 12 inches above the top canopy using easily adjustable light holders.

the sun shines.

At my home, I have a small greenhouse surrounded on three sides by building walls. Light is admitted only from the top and the southwest-facing side.

The greenhouse is kept moist to provide the right environment for tropical orchids and for overwintering plumerias: the plants that produce Hawaii's fragrant lei flowers. The sun heats the greenhouse naturally to the high 70s daily. A CO_2 generator controlled by a thermostat doesn't allow the temperature to slide below 60 degrees in the evenings, within the tropical plan s' comfort range and also very pleasant for young marijuana plants.

As you can imagine, the amount of light ente ing the greenhouse is nominal, especially this time of year when the sun sits low on the horizon. A quartet of 55-watt T5 fluorescents hang over the orchids, and another 55-watt foursome and a 100-watt fluorescent hang over the marijuana plants, supplementing sun and ambient light when it's most intense.

My plan is to grow on a table, below the canopy of the plumeria, which are deciduous in this environment—they lose a lot of their leaves if the temperature falls into the low 50s. Some light will get through, but it needs to be supplemented. I decided to use a 75-watt white diode LED fixture that's installed to hang below the plumeria, only 12 inches over the canopy.

I bought three clones—Fire OG, Purple Kush, and Candyland—from a local dispensary and kept them for two days on a table that received daylight in the kitchen. The lights were turned on throughout the day and evening so the plants were kept in a vegetative state.

The clones had been rooted in 2-inch rockwool cubes. I planted them in soft-cloth containers that I had used briefly during a previous experiment. Wicks had already been installed in

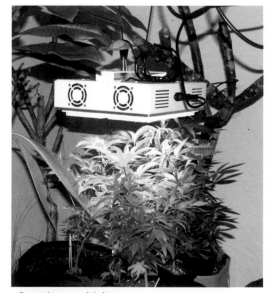

Greenhouse with its new cannabis additions.

the 5-gallon bags, and they were already filled with barely used planting mix. This certainly reduced time spent planting. I positioned each cube so its top was slightly raised from the planting mix and the stem would stay dry, discouraging pathogens. Then I watered the mix with a dilute vegetative fertilizer to help bond it with the cube.

I placed a Styrofoam board on the cold cement floor as a temperature barrier. Then I placed the planted containers on the board and turned on the LEDs. Unlike the other lights in the greenhouse, these lights will remain on continuously for a few weeks to encourage plant growth and to keep the plants in the vegetative stage, rather than switching to flowering, which is induced by long nights. In a few weeks the lights will be turned back and the plants will flower. When it's clear, I plan to take the plants out into direct sunlight.

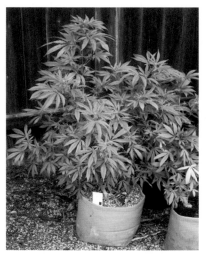

This Juicy Fruit is the largest plant.

MOVING THE PLANTS OUTDOORS

A month later, in mid-February, the cold days of January were past. The temperature was not likely to go below 45 degrees at night, with daytime temperatures in the high 60s, and occasionally the low 70s. It was time to move the plants outside to bask in the sun. With sunlight on them, leaf temperature stays warmer than the surrounding air. The photosynthetic rate increases as the temperatures rise.

Outdoors, the plants joined an older plant, transplanted into a 5-gallon soft-sided container around January 25. I placed a sealed electric heater set at 72 degrees at the bottom of the container to keep the roots warm and protected from the January chill. That helped it survive the coolest temperatures. The plant was purchased at a dispensary as a 3-foot branched adolescent still in the vegetative stage.

As soon as it was placed outside, it began to switch to flowering growth because the dark period was more than 13 hours and would remain longer than 12 hours until the vernal equinox on March 22. The former adolescent was now in its fourth week of flowering. Its growth had been delayed a bit by cool weather, but with the warmer days the flowers' growth would spurt.

The three clones transplanted into 5-gallon soft-sided containers spent the month of January sitting on a table in the greenhouse, receiving ambient light as well as continuous light from a white LED fixture. They filled out a bit, but the light kept the plants very dense, without much intermodal length. So they were only about 18 inches tall.

Shortly after planting, a friend asked me to hold a couple of clones until he left for home, upstate. I placed them on top of two of the 5-gallon containers. However, he left town without retrieving the plants. I also left. When I returned ten days later, the roots had grown into the larger container, so I left them there.

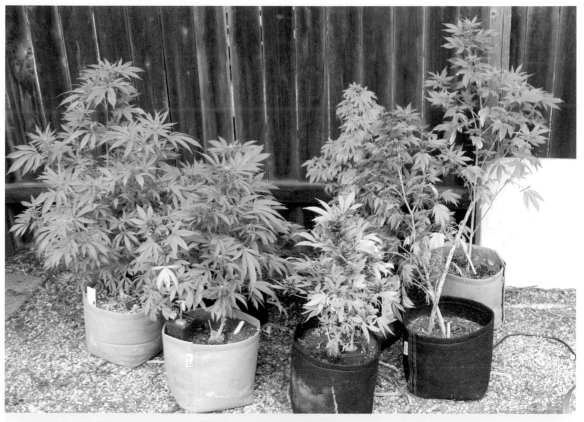

Notice the differences between varieties in shape and color. Growing small plants is a good way to determine potency and effects, comparative yield, growth patterns and other varietal variations.

WHY ARE THERE SO MANY DIFFERENCES IN VARIETIES?

Plants of the same population from higher latitudes have a lot of variability. These include Southern Africans, Northern Mexicans, and indicas. Cannabsi within these groups look slightly different from each other and have different maturities and potency. The ratio of THC (the psychoactive ingredient) also varies. The differences in native climate makes low-latitude populations more homogeneous and high-latitude populations heterogeneous.

Plant varieties originating in lower latitudes have less variation within their population. There is little change of weather in more tropical areas, where every year tends to resemble the last. In temperate climates, by contrast, there can be wide variability—one year may be cold and rainy, the next hot and dry.

The wide selection of characteristics in northern-latitude varieties means that some individual plants will thrive no matter what conditions occur in a particular season. Most varieties available today are hybrids of these types, and bred to have the best characteristics of each. Most of the varieties offered today are many hybridizations away from the original landraces from which they started. They have been totally domesticated to modern standards.

Before I filled them with coir-based planting mix all the containers were outfitted with wicks made from 3/8-inch (1 cm) braided nylon rope that hangs down from the holes at the bottom of each pot. When the ends are placed in a reservoir, they transport water up to the planting mix using capillary action. The reservoir and supports will soon be installed. One advantage is that only the reservoir has to be kept filled, so chores are reduced. In addition, the containers water themselves as needed.

The plants spent their first day under the sun on February 12. Tomorrow the sun rises at 7:01 a.m. and sets at 5:45 p.m., providing 10 hours and 44 minutes of light. The dark period is 13 hours and 16 minutes. The long dark period will promote the fast switch from vegetative to flowering mode.

MORE PLANTS JOIN THE FUN AND THE GARDEN GROWS

After setting up the garden, I spent some time with my tiny plants that, at nature's urging (in the form of a long dark period nightly), would soon experience the change to reproductive mode, flowering. They were so small and took up so little space. Each would produce only a small amount of genuine California outdoor bud, and they needed such little maintenance—just watering with bloom formula a couple of times weekly during warm weather, and once weekly or less during cooler periods.

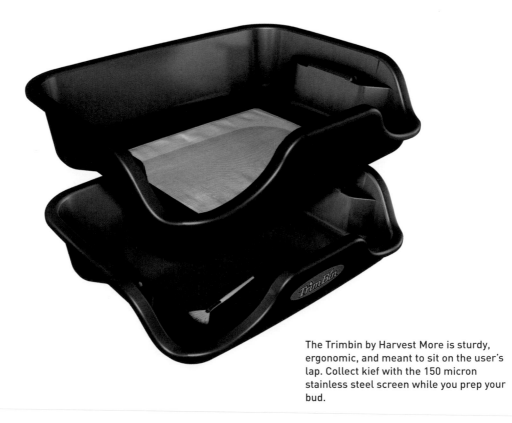

The Trimbin by Harvest More is sturdy, ergonomic, and meant to sit on the user's lap. Collect kief with the 150 micron stainless steel screen while you prep your bud.

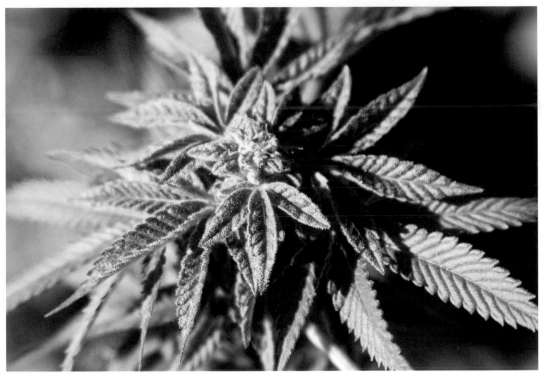

This Girl Scout Cookies bud is about halfway through flowering. Although small, it took little effort and will be quite potent.

While contemplating the garden, I decided to adopt more plants to join the few already there. My friend George had a teenage Purple Pineapple that he was going to clone out when he had the chance, but he saw those tiny plants and felt that they needed company. Then I decided to check out the teenager situation at one of the local dispensaries, twice. Each time there was only one suitable plant. I was looking for plants that had at least a few strong branches that would support cola growth.

After I brought the plants home, I transplanted them from the 6-inch 1-quart pots to 5-gallon containers. Then I set them out to meet their new friends and to introduce them to their new source of energy—El Sol. Although it was a bright sunny day, the light in February in the San Francisco Bay Area is not so intense that plants need a gentle introduction using shading or protection of some sort. They were placed under full sun immediately.

As expected, the plants started to flower soon after they were put outdoors. Three weeks into their flower growth, with another five to go, harvest was on track for the first week in April. I didn't expect a large harvest, but it's always nice to have some ounces of fresh outdoor growth to use in the spring.

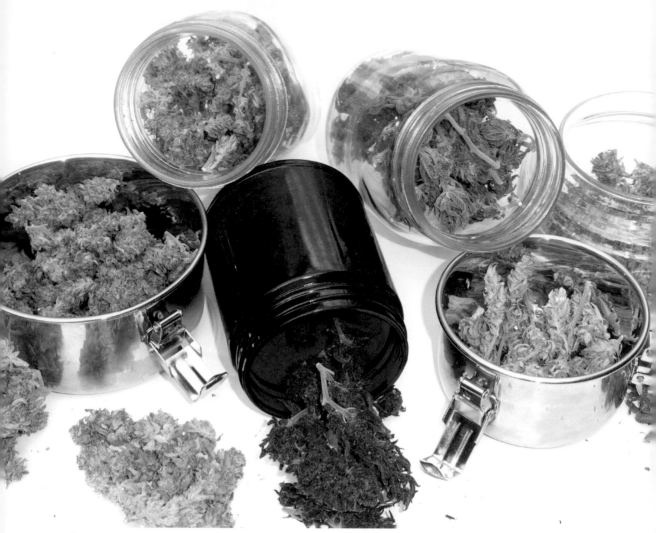

There were eight varieties in the garden. Here's their group graduation photo. This material will be destroyed using controlled burns.

HARVESTING MY HOME GARDEN

I was away from late February to early April. But the die was cast. The plants had already been transplanted into their final containers: 3- or 5-gallon soft-sided pots. They were set out in the sunniest part of the garden at the beginning of February in the middle of winter, when the nights are long. Growing under long nights, the plants started to flower within a week of placement. They were fed flowering formula fertilizer at half strength weekly until March 10. Then they were given just plain water. There was enough residual fertilizer in the soil to keep them going for a few weeks, and then the plants used the excess they were carrying internally.

March 21 is the date of the vernal equinox—day and night are equal—the first day of spring. Between March 22 and April 10 the nights were growing shorter, but the day's increasing length did not affect the plants' flowering. Most of the plants in the garden would initiate flowering under only 10 hours of uninterrupted darkness, and the increasing light never crossed that critical time period of 14 hours of light.

Light provides the energy for photosynthesis, the process in which plants split water (H_2O) into its constituent elements, hydrogen and oxygen. The oxygen is released into the atmosphere. The hydrogen is combined with carbon dioxide (CO_2) to form sugar, which the plants use for energy and for tissue building. With more intense light, plants have more energy to grow bigger, faster.

During February and March, the sun's light is not very intense, so the plants receive less light energy than in summer—less energy to use for growth. In addition, each day stays warm just until the sun sets. Cool temperatures slow growth. So the buds are smaller than they would be with a summer crop or if the garden had been placed under plastic to keep the plants warmer. One advantage to the February start is that the intensity of the light increases as the buds grow.

On April 10, the buds looked ripe. They weren't big, but they were covered with trichomes, and the stigmas had all dried red-brown or purple. The buds were ready to be cut and dried. The plants were easily cut by bending the stems until they snapped. Then scissors were used to complete the separation. The buds were placed on a tray and carried to the drying area, where they were hung from nylon fishing line inside an unused grow tent.

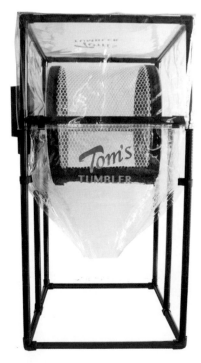
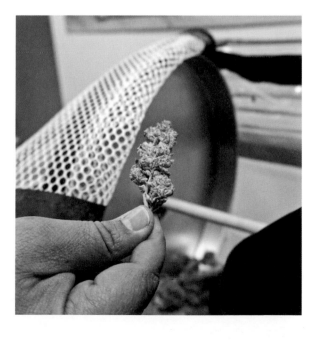

Tom's most popular tumbler, the TTT 1900 system, trims, separates, and collects keif without the use of blades. The trimming rate is 1 to 2 pounds every 3-5 minutes and replicates hand trimmed quality after brief touch up. The gentle action of the buds rubbing against each other instead of blades is what makes Tom's Tumblers superior to other technologies. Trichomes and terpenes are minimally affected and dry trimming ensures a strong aroma. Tom's Tumbler TTT 1900 is a great solution for small and medium-sized growers.

DRY, TRIM, ENJOY

It had been more than two weeks since I hung the plants to dry in a tent in an unheated room. The temperature range in the room was 55 to 70 degrees, and the humidity was usually in the 50% range. An oscillating fan on low speed was placed a few feet away from the tent so the plants were constantly buffeted by a slight breeze.

I had been traveling during the time the plants were drying and curing, and by the time I got back, they were ready to be manicured.

One indication of their readiness was the break test. Small branches near the bud broke with a snap rather than bending when twisted. This is a good sign that the buds are dry enough.

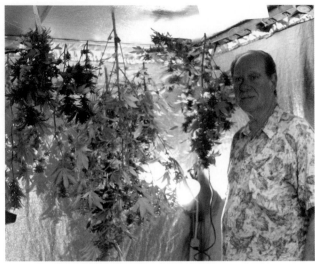

Here I am with the harvest that I hung in a vacant grow tent. The temperature in the room varies between 60°F and 75°F. The plants should be dried and cured in about two weeks. Then I will manicure, package, and utilize the buds.

Another was that the buds had only a bit of spring when squeezed, but they weren't crisp either, which is a sign of overdrying.

While manicuring can be an enjoyable way to spend some time, especially if you're in a social

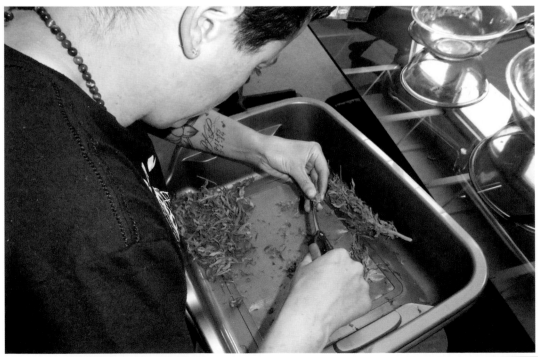

Expert trimmer Stacy at work.

circle enjoying the harvest with good company, I decided to take a friend up on her offer to manicure the plants in return for some of the bounty.

When I harvested for the first time in April, I left some of the smaller, immature buds on the plants, hoping that the plants would regenerate and move back into vegetative growth. They would produce leaves rather than buds, and then in the fall they would flower again, allowing a second harvest.

However, the buds that were left

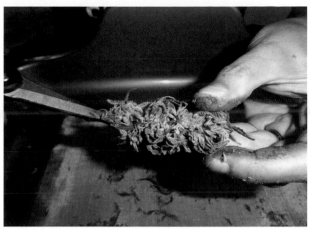

All the buds were heavily coated with trichomes.

actually grew a little once they started getting nutrients that were going to the top buds, and then they matured. I'm planning on harvesting them tomorrow, followed by a second round of drying.

I hope that after this harvest, the May nights will finally be short enough to induce the plants to go back into vegetative growth.

Here are the stats on the plants:

Name	Weight
1. Juicy Fruit	22 grams
2. Juicy Fruit 2	58 grams
3. Candy Land	44 grams
4. Girl Scout Cookies	55 grams
5. Fire OG	22 grams
6. Purple Pineapple	32 grams
7. Purple Kush	25 grams
8. Killa Watt	52 grams
Total:	310 grams

When I showed some of the buds to visitors, they were unimpressed. The buds were small, and although fragrant and heady, they weren't very tight. However, I was more than satisfied because this was a winter crop started in February and harvested in April. I didn't expect big buds, but I did produce a decent harvest using the winter sun.

No one complained about the buds when rolled. They were potent and had high levels of terpenes despite the early season harvest. Perhaps the cool temperatures preserved more of the terpenes that were produced.

Chapter 14

Fall Quickie Garden

Covers:
- How to plant late in the season for a fall harvest

Early in October a friend gave me a couple of plants to test the toxicity of an organic pesticide. The toxicity results were negative, which was positive. The pesticide didn't affect the plants negatively. Both specimens were healthy.

Now I was left with the two "3x Crazy" plants. The plants were receiving a little less than 12 hours of natural light daily, with early morning and sundown in shade. A month later they would be receiving only 10.75 hours daily. Of course, under this regimen the plants went into flower immediately.

The weather was warm during the entire month of October, so I decided to keep the plants outside and let them flower under the short days of autumn. The plants were in small containers, so it was easy to move them around the yard three times daily as the sunny area shifted.

By early November the nighttime temperature had dipped into the high 40s. I decided on a routine change. Instead of leaving the plants out at night, I carried them into the greenhouse and set up supplemental light from a 1000-watt HPS light. The routine went as follows.

7 A.M. Plants are indoors. Light goes on.

10 A.M. Plants are carried outside to sunny section of yard as long as it's not cloudy or rainy and the temperature is above 68°. Otherwise, the plants are kept indoors with the light on. If outside, plants are moved various times during the day to keep them in sunny locations.

4:30 P.M. Plants are moved back to the greenhouse. Lights are on.

6 P.M. Lights go off.

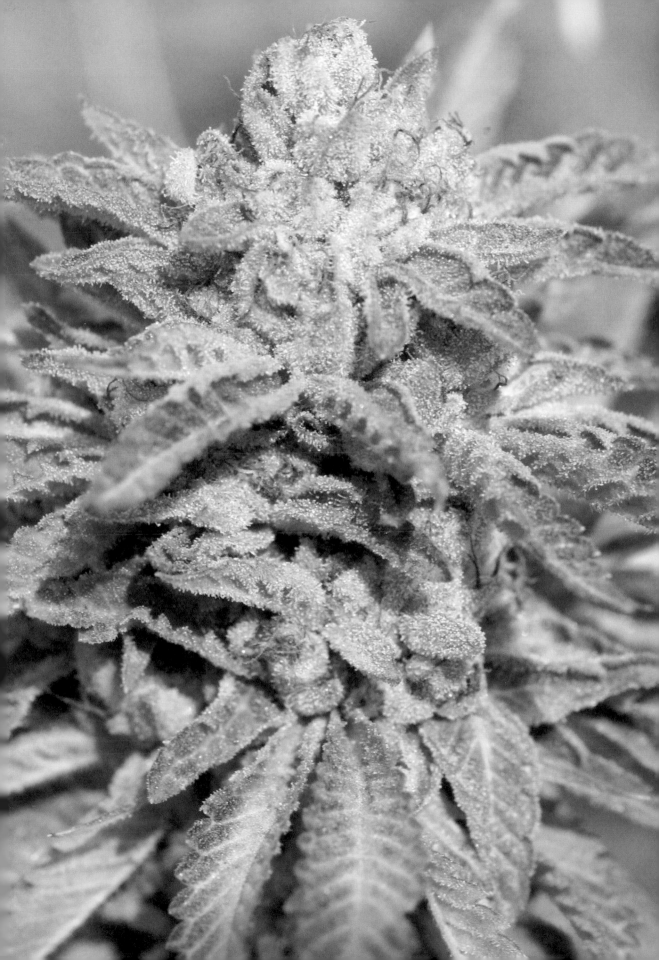

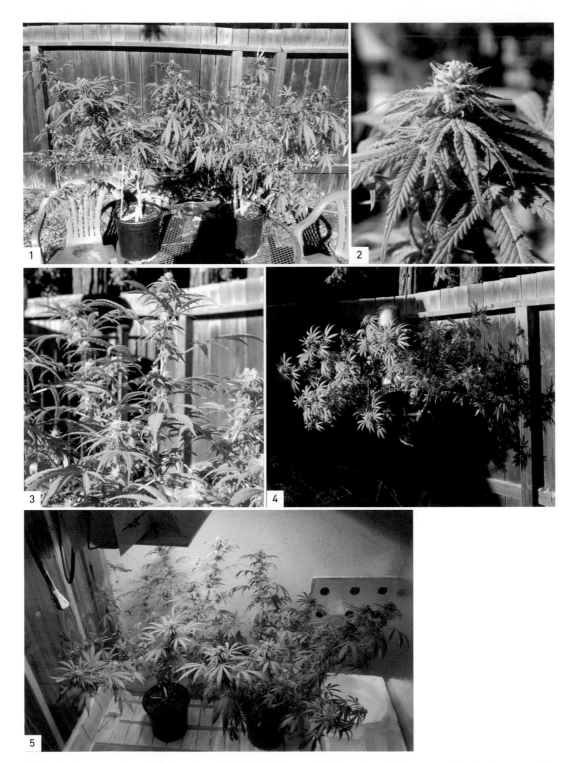

1. The plants were placed outdoors in early October. One month later, in early November, the plants were midway through flowering.   2. Close-up of one of the small flowers.

3. Each branch was developing into a cola.   4. Plants being moved to a sunny area of the yard.

5. Plants basking under 1000 watt lamp.With colder nights and dimming sun the plants started receiving enhanced care: supplemental lighting in the morning and evening and shelter from the cold.

On most days the HPS lamp was used for only 4.5 hours, and on cold, foggy, or rainy days, which are infrequent here in Northern California, the light was on all day. The plants stay inside when I'm away from home.

Using this technique, I was minimizing energy use, but still getting light to the plants. I realize that in some areas of the country it's just too cold to put the plants out anytime during the fall going into winter. The light is just too dim. Still, you might be able to use a south-facing window, a skylight, or a greenhouse to supply supplemental light to meet the plants' light requirements.

The 400-watt HPS lamp hung from a light mover was set to move back and forth about 2 feet, covering the length of the garden with light. In November it was still often sunny and warm enough for the plants to go outdoors for some natural sunlight between 10 a.m. and 4 p.m. When they returned to the greenhouse, they received another 2 hours of light from the HPS lamp.

Toward the end of the month the weather turned cloudy and chilly. Then the plants enjoyed the cozy greenhouse, which was kept at a minimum temperature of 60 degrees day and night.

Fifty-five days passed since the plants started their short photoperiod, and they were ready to harvest. The buds are small but are covered with trichomes and have an intense floral/pineapple/diesel odor.

I picked the plants late in November and hung them to dry and cure in an unheated indoor space. At that time of the year, the temperature varies between the low 50s and high 60s. The humidity varies between 43% and 54%, with an average at just about 50%. These are ideal conditions for a long, slow dry and cure.

The low temperature keeps the terpenes from evaporating. Terpenes, the

The Hang. The two plants will now begin the monthlong drying/curing process. They'll be manicured after that.

odor molecules that give all marijuana varieties their particular "personalities," are essential oils. Many of them are volatile at room temperature, so they're often lost in the dry, transport, or storage phases. The low temperature in the drying space keeps them from evaporating, and they will lend their odor and activity to the smoke or vapor.

Rather than mess with cutting these small plants into branches, I hung them uncut with all their leaves on. They were aged for several weeks after they dried, with cool temperatures and 50% humidity. During this time they lost their harshness, becoming a smoother smoke. Then I manicured them and placed them in a steel metal container made for that purpose, which comes with a holder for a Boveda pad that stabilizes moisture, keeping the buds fresh.

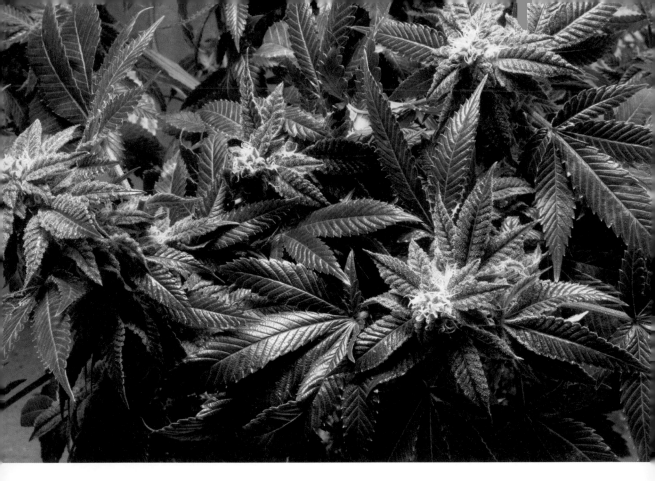

Chapter 15

Winter Garden

Covers:
- Using natural and supplemental light
- Growing with the changing seasons

MY INDOOR WINTER GARDEN

The garden has been empty for about two months, and I'm restarting. It's the first week of January, and the days are short, only 9 hours of daylight, much of it dim.

My plan was to visit a local dispensary and buy about thirty clones. I would have repotted them into 8-inch containers and vegetate them for a week before forcing the instant sea of green to flower. However, I saw a beautiful Shark Shock plant, mostly indica, with parentage of White Widow and

Skunk #1, at the shop. I decided to buy that instead.

The plant is 24 inches tall with a canopy that spreads out 39 inches in a great circle. It had a lot of side branches that I trimmed off and will use for cloning.

It was growing in a 2½-gallon container, and the roots were lightly circling the sides. The plant was placed in its new home, a 5-gallon container. The old container was a little shorter than the new one, so I added enough mix to the bottom of the new one, to allow the plant stem to sit at the same level, and filled the sides with planting mix. I placed the container in a tray to catch excess water, keeping the space neat.

Water that drains into the tray is soon soaked up by the container. I placed the tray on a Styrofoam sheet to block the cold concrete floor from draining heat from the container and cooling the roots.

The plant basks in my greenhouse under a 600-watt HPS lamp. It receives several hours of direct sunlight as well as ambient light. As the sun's position changes seasonally, the greenhouse will receive more sunlight, boosting growth as the flowers are in their last stages of ripening.

I kept the plant growing vegetatively, rather than flowering, for two weeks by interrupting the dark period. This was accomplished with a 5-minute burst of light from a 40-watt warm-white compact fluorescent every 2 hours during the dark period. It was fertilized once using a 7-9-5 one-part complete vegetative formula fertilizer diluted to 700 ppm.

A timer turns the light on at 6 a.m., just before dawn now, and it goes off at 6 p.m., slightly after sunset.

The greenhouse is kept at 62 degrees at night using a gas heater, with thermostat attached, and a backup electric heater set at 60 degrees. A minimum temperature of 70 degrees is maintained during the day.

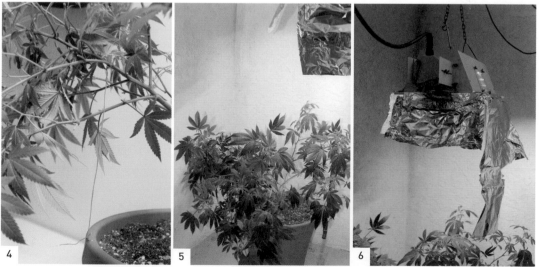

1 Branches were "trained" lower using a horticultural twist-tie.
2. In the greenhouse the plant receives both natural and generated lighting.
3. Aluminum foil was taped to reflector to direct more light to the plant.

TRANSPLANTING THE SHARK SHOCK

Two weeks after the plant moved into its 5-gallon container, the regulatory lights that flashed each evening were turned off and the formula was changed to a one-part bloom formula, 3-12-6. Five days later the first flowers appeared. A few days after, they were covering all the branches.

Soon after transplanting I began "training" the plant. I wanted it to completely fill the 4′ × 4′ canopy, 16 square feet, and to encourage the large branches capable of producing large buds.

On its own, Shark Shock grows a large main stem with big buds and smaller side branches that produce smaller buds. Clipping the main bud early results in several main branches that will yield more than the large single bud.

The plant had been clipped when it was young, so it had branched out somewhat. I started by "horizontalizing" the branches: bending them so they were parallel to the floor rather than growing up. I bent some down and held them in place using twist ties attached to little holes drilled at the container top to hold them in place. Others were bent and held in place using crutches. At the same time, understory and small branches were removed, leaving only large bud sites. The small branches and leaves that were shaded would be lackluster producers, and they cost the plant energy because it doesn't get light.

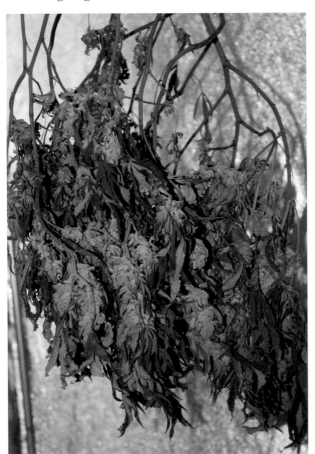

The plant hung in the tent for almost a month.

Horizontalizing the plant, similar to scrogging, but without the screen, produces a higher yield because the plant covers a much large canopy.

The results were apparent thirty days later. All the buds were at about the same height, so they didn't block each other's light. The entire canopy was filled with bud sites, and the flowering formula encouraged new bud formation. The increasing intensity of the sunlight and ambient light as spring draws closer also helped increase the growth rate.

HARVESTING AND TRIMMING

Once the flowers appeared, I fed the plant with a set of six fertilizers and supplements for blooming. The plant showed signs of overfertilization, so I waited several weeks to feed it again.

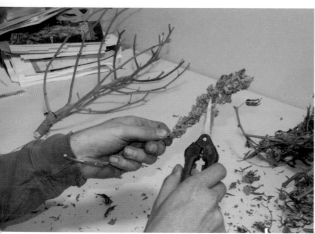
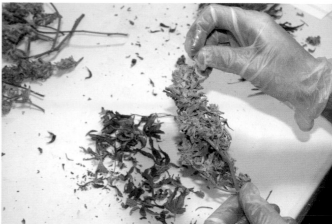

Buds were trimmed of leaves and removed from cola.

The plant flowers were tight. I hung the whole plant in an empty gro-tent inside a room that stays at 50–60% humidity and a temperature below 70 degrees.

The room stayed within an ideal range of temperature and humidity. Rather than separate the drying and curing stages with clear delineation, I just let the plant hang and slowly reach maturity.

A month went by, and it was time to take down the plant and manicure it.

Manicuring was easy. First, the colas were removed from the branches using a pair of garden clippers. Then, the buds were manicured while remaining on the cola.

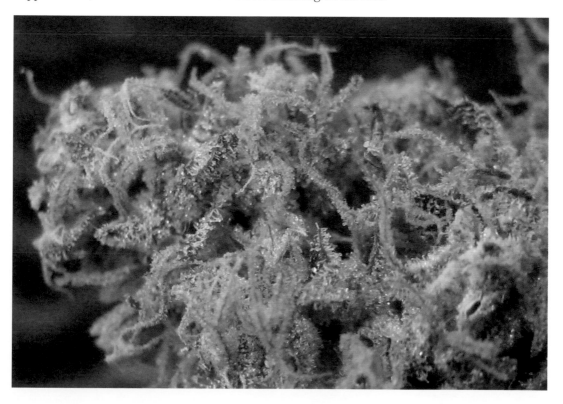

Chapter 16

A Three-Month Spring/Summer Garden

Covers:
- Planting to maximize light
- Mobile gardens
- Outdoors or in a greenhouse? Both!

I started preparing my three-part spring garden in April.

STARTING THE GARDEN
GROUP 1: SMALL PLANTS

Group 1 consists of four plants that I was given as small rooted cuttings. They'd been growing for six weeks. I transplanted them into 6-inch containers shortly after I received them and had them growing under continuous light from a 400-watt LED for about three weeks. Then I moved them into my small greenhouse. Two weeks after that, the roots had filled the container and left their cramped quarters for roomier 5-gallon containers. Ten days later, the plants had doubled in size.

They were all healthy and seemed to be enjoying their special treatment. In the early morning they hung out in the greenhouse. Shortly after dawn, at about 6 a.m., a 320-watt induction fluorescent started supplementing the early morning light. This continued for about 4 hours. At 10 a.m. they were carried outside and placed in the sun close to a wall that reflects the light back at them. To

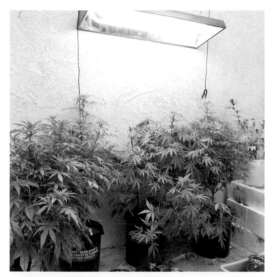

In the greenhouse the plants get light in the late afternoon and early evening.

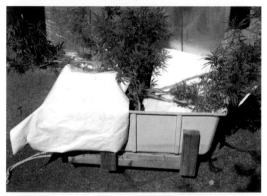

The plants in the unit are basking in the sun.

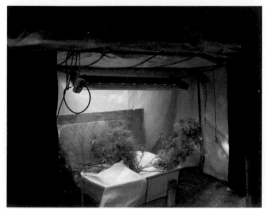

They are wheeled into the tent to have cozy nights and a bit of light.

amplify the effect, I use Styrofoam boards placed at an angle, aimed at the plants.

Later in the day that area becomes shady, so the plants are moved a few feet away to another section of the garden that gets afternoon sun. Then, around 6 p.m., they're placed back in the greenhouse and receive supplemental light until 8 p.m., close to sunset.

To keep the plants from flowering and to have them respond quickly when I change the cycle to flowering in late June, I break up the dark period periodically. At night the plants receive light from two 4-foot fluorescents for 2 minutes every hour from 9 p.m. until 5 a.m. I accomplished this using a repeating two-dial timer. I set the first dial for the amount of time I want the light to work, and the other dial for the amount of time it takes to complete the cycle. Then I plug that timer into a 24-hour timer set in the "on" position only during the night.

RESCUING A FEW MORE NEEDY PLANTS

Sometimes I use plants to test pesticides for plant toxicity. I had this group of plants—three small ones and two larger ones—that was used for testing, and after the tests were over, the plants were neglected. There they were, sitting in a tent with lights shining but no water for several weeks. By the time I rediscovered them, they were three quarters dead. To save them, I started by giving them some water for a few days, until they recovered from the drought, then I started bringing them outside during the day.

The next week I set them up in the new moveable space they now share. I started with a moving dolly and secured a half-inch-thick piece of plywood 2 × 4 to it with screws. Next, I attached a rope to the plywood on one of the

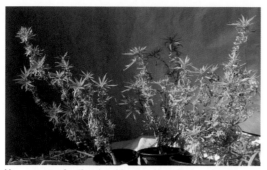

You can see by the dead leaves that these plants weren't doing well. They are making a good recovery.

narrow sides so the unit could easily be pulled. On the dolly I placed a 9-inch-deep 2' × 4' horticultural tray set up with wick systems made from 3/8-inch braided nylon rope. Then I filled the tray with a mixture of enriched potting soil, coir fiber, and homemade compost from kitchen wastes and plant material consisting mostly of oak leaves.

I set the long-suffering plants in place. The two larger ones were placed sideways in the tray with the roots at the bottom of the container against the tray side buried halfway, with the other half making a mound. Each root mound was covered with half a potting container cut with a small electric saw. The plants' stems were long enough to leave the center of the tray bare. That's where I planted the three small specimens, upright.

These plants had a regimen similar to the other plants. They spent evenings in a little tent lit with 200 watts of fluorescent light, and their days basking in the sun.

Within two weeks after transplanting, the sideways plants made the adjustment. They came back to life.

HORIZONTAL TRANSPLANTING

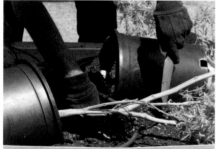

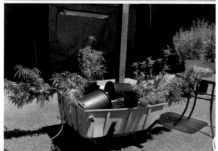

SUMMER HEAT AND SOME NEW ADDITIONS TO MY MOBILE GARDEN

June 22, the first day of summer and the longest day of the year, is when the sun's rays shine most directly on us, so the light is most intense. The bright light was great for the plants in the three sections of my garden. All of them had a growth spurt and were extremely healthy.

The 2 × 4, 9-inch-deep tray held five plants. A month later the five plants are 2 feet tall and have been growing more than an inch a day. Just yesterday I changed their regimen from vegetative to flowering. Each evening I placed the cart in its own little growth chamber, with about 200 watts of fluorescent light so that the plant was kept lit continuously.

I started wheeling the cart into the unlit chamber sometime after dusk, which occurs around 9 p.m. The plants stayed there until 9 a.m., for a dark period of 12 hours each evening. The plants had a few flowers, but in about two months the colas would be ready to harvest.

The plants were wheeled into a dark tent area each day for light deprivation and harvested on July 24, after fifty-six days of flowering. The branches were cut and hung in a slow dry/cure.

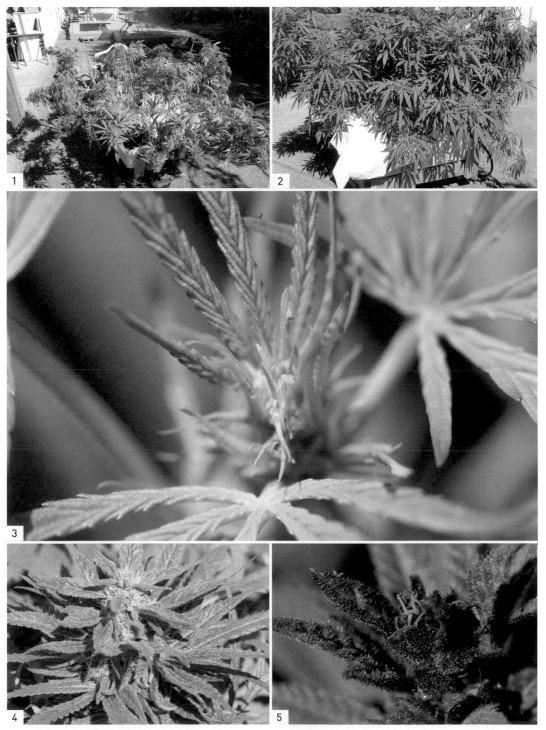

1. The plants on wheels basking in the sun. The stem was placed horizontally so the branches are growing vertically.   2. Early flowering of the plants on wheels. The plants have been in flowering regimen for 4 days.
3. Plants in 8" containers. Tops of half of them were clipped on June19. All are indicas from the same group. They have thick stems, and wide leaves with purple tones.   4. Close-up of the bud; it should be ready in 4 or 5 weeks.   5. Close-up of pollinated Purple Citrus

GROUP 2: CLONES

Group 2, in my three-part garden, consisted of four plants grown from clones, including a Shark Shock and an ER Superbud, and two dwarfed plants identified as Purple Dream but perhaps are another variety. These plants had been flowering for a while, but I was afraid that they would switch back to vegetative growth. So I also sheltered them in darkness each evening, using the same regimen as for the first group. A month later they were harvested and drying.

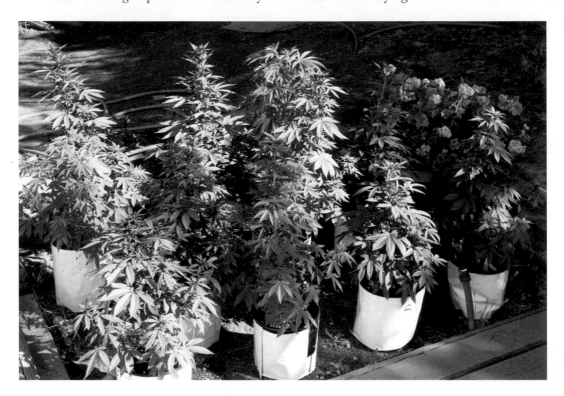

GROUP 3: COMPOST RESCUES

Group 3 started out as ten volunteers in my compost pile. Luckily for them, a member of the plant rescue society saw them around June 1 and placed them in 4-inch pots. They soon outgrew the containers and were placed in 6-inch containers. They were replanted again, two in early July, into 8-inch containers. The plants were all indicas, and all seemed closely related. They had broad leaves and short internodes, and were beginning to get purple. It looked like a fine strain. The plants were now 10–14 inches tall and growing quickly under a natural daylight and indoor light regimen. Eventually, I identified them as variations on a wide-leaved Purple Pineapple, and all had similar characteristics.

The ten plants, all female, started flowering shortly after germinating. It was apparent that the seeds were strays generated by the Purple Pineapple mother and unknown male pollen, perhaps a hidden hermaphrodite in the last generation of PPs. They finished flowering on about July 27.

I performed several demonstration experiments on this group of plants. First, because they

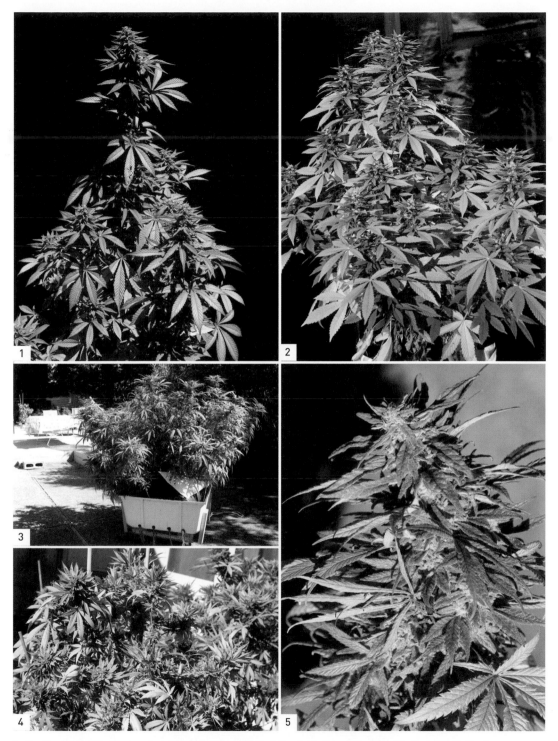

1. Unclipped Purple Pineapple had a large top bud that dominated growth. The side bud didn't develop very much. 2. Top clipped Purple Pineapple's central bud did not dominate growth. Instead, without inhibition from hormones produced by top bud, the side buds grew out producing a bigger yield. 3. The 2' x 4' tray held 5 Blue Dream plants. Buds and foliage covered the entire container then spread out further. 4. The four plants started flowering early because they were placed outdoors in early spring when the natural light period was too short to maintain vegetative growth. 5. Bud of Blackberry Fire plant is ready to harvest.

started flowering early, they grew to a controlled size. My goal was to demonstrate that cannabis could be grown as small row plants, making cultivation easier with conventional farming techniques, rather than as large plants more reminiscent of orchards.

In another experiment I paired plants about equal in growth and pruned their top half so that some were cut and some were not. You can see the difference in their growth. The uncut plant grew a larger central bud at the expense of side growth. The cut plants produced several branches that held more buds than the uncut plants. These plants were ready to harvest about ninety days after germination. They were cut and hung whole to dry as well. They'll all be dried and cured next month. Then they'll be manicured.

TRIMMING, DRYING AND CURING MY SUMMER HARVEST

Early this summer I used light deprivation, providing 12 hours of uninterrupted darkness to induce flowering. The plants were all harvested over a two-week period beginning the last week of July.

After being cut, large branches or whole plants were hung to dry in a cool cellar-type space that mostly maintained temperatures in the high 60s and had about 50% relative humidity.

They remained unmanicured as they dried and cured over two months, until there was time to separate the buds from the stem and then to unveil the bud from its shield of trim leaves.

The buds are perfectly dry: moist enough to retain sponginess and to return to shape after they're squeezed, rather than too dry, when they just crack and crisp into little pieces. At the same time, the little stem that holds the buds to the cola cracks rather than bending. The dry trim leaves peel away from the tight bud nuggets to reveal crystal-like, perfectly mature buds that have retained their odor.

First, we trimmed the cured bud, removing any fan leaves that were left, and then we started removing the trim leaves. We soon realized that we were too bored, and it seemed like too much effort to continue the task. So we made a strategic decision: to leave the trim leaves on the buds and to remove them only as the buds are removed from their storage container to be destroyed using a controlled burn. The buds were quickly placed into jars and metal storage containers. They'll be stored in the refrigerator.

Because the bud was slow-dried and cured in a cool space, a high percentage of terpenes were retained, and the bud has great odors. I'm toking on some Blue Dream as I'm writing this, and even though I'm outdoors, the floral odor surrounds me.

The SuperBud is more complex, expressing a spicy highlight that rises above a more sedate stoniness, including a sweet candy taste but spicy odors. The effect is both relaxing and invigorating.

The Chocolate Tonic is very earthy. Its odor is sort of like a medical tonic. The effect is mellow, sedating, and calming. A nice variety for relaxing, but not zoning out.

The Blackberry Fire's taste and odor was very generic. The high crept up slowly into a sativa space that conserved energy and encouraged inquiry.

The summer crop has been processed and is sitting in the refrigerator and freezer waiting for eventual destruction. It offers a wide choice of highs and will create many altered states among

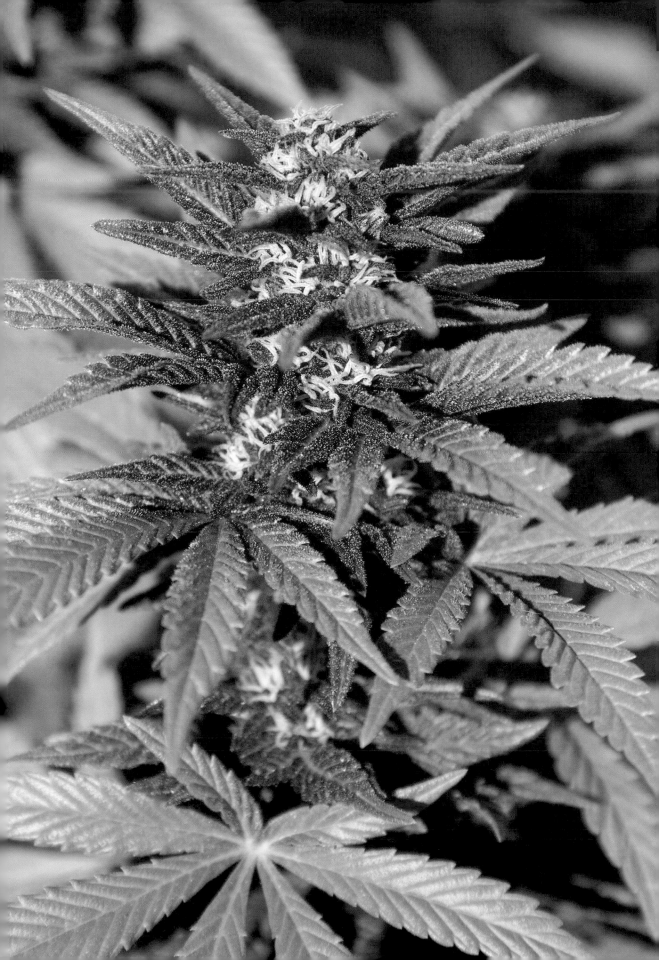

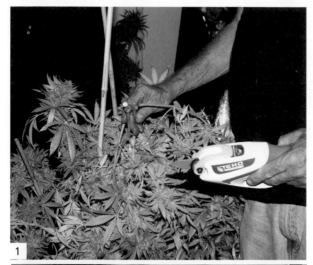

1

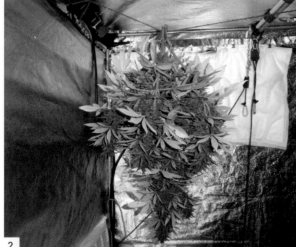

2

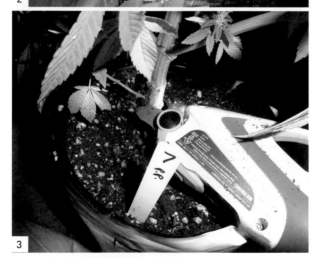

3

friends and family.

Harvest is celebrated all over the world. Yet our urban connection to the bounties of nature is usually a short one, just to the store or restaurant. Cannabis is the only plant some people grow, and that's fitting, because it might be the first plant grown by humans. So when cultivators toke up, we rediscover the wonders of nature.

And if you're a cultivator, you know that yours is the best in the world. And I would not dispute that. Using the grass that you grew provides a pleasure that cannot be matched by gift or purchased weed. It's a connection to the wheel of life.

Enjoy.

1. Trimming some Blue Dream for immediate use.
2. Hanging fresh buds from the tray.
3. Cutting stem using electric cutter.
4. Hung plants

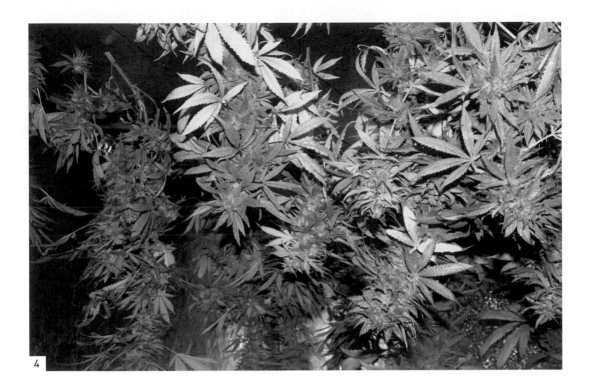

4

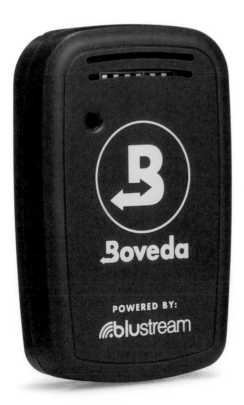

The Boveda Butler is the most precise humidity management system for curing and storing. Protect your terpenes from evaporation and ensure optimal long-term storage conditions for your cannabis.

Ask Ed

COMMON DRYING AND HARVESTING QUESTIONS

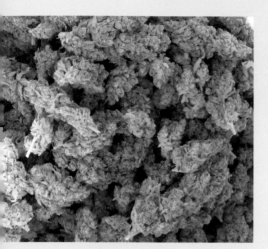

DRYING

I cure the buds at between 18 to 20°C at 50 percent for the first three days. What should I do to dry it at after that?

Raise the temperature a few degrees, no higher than 22°C, and lower the humidity to 40 to 45 percent. Keep the buds in the drying zone until the tiny sticks in the buds snap. This happens when they have only 10 to 8 percent moisture. Only then are they ready for packaging.

Don't let them get drier or they won't be suitable for smoking.

POOR ROOTS AND SMALL HARVESTS

I have been growing in coco for several years now. The quality has been good but the yields have been small. The roots are small and poorly developed.

The garden has CO_2. The room stays 22° to 23° C when the lights are on and I don't overwater. I keep the nutrient solution at 1600 ppm including the 450-ppm naturally occurring in my tap water.

Marijuana is a short-day plant, which means that its flowering cycle is based on the number of

hours of uninterrupted darkness it receives. It measures light and darkness based on red and far-red light and, to a much lesser effect, based on blue light.

Short-day plants are not affected by green light in regard to the flowering cycle, so it is safe to leave a green light on during the flowering period. Both LED and fluorescent green lights do not emit red light so they are excellent sources of green light.

GROWING KILLER WEED

Whats the most important factor in growing killer weed? Would it be soil, temperature, nutrients, or something else?

The most important factor that affects the quality of the weed you are growing is the plant's genetics. No matter how well a plant is grown, it can only reach its genetic potential. The cheapest way to improve your garden is to find better varieties.

Environmental conditions enhance the potential of your crop, or rather; they can hinder your plants from reaching their full potential if the plants' basic needs are not met. Light, water nutrients, CO_2 and temperature are the limiting factors.

HARVEST RAIN

Three days left to harvest moon, but we have rain forecast. I'm worried about mold. Should the ladies go or stay three more days?

_____

The plants aren't going to grow or mature much during cool, cloudy and rainy weather. So delaying harvest won't help them much.

SEED TO FLOWER

I'd like to report on a little experiment I performed.

I tried the seed to flower method used in the book "Let's Grow Pound". The area was 2 meters square lit by two 400w HPS lamps. I used 12 2-liter containers each sown with 3 Blueberry seeds by DJ Short so I could eliminate the males.

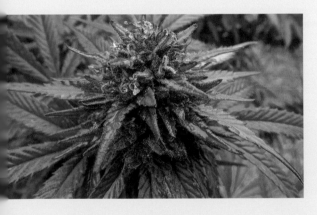

The seeds were germinated directly in the soil under 12 hours of light. 14 days after the seeds had germinated, I could distinguish sex. Only about a third of the plants were males so I was left with two plants in most containers.

During week 4 all the plants began to flower profusely and they ripened between weeks 9 and 11. The yield was about 700g, averaging about a bit more than 30 grams per plant.

The next time I used fewer plants to see how they would fill the room using a cross of Purple Tops x Anesthesia. This time I used a single 400W HPS light and seeded four 2 liter pots, using soil amended with mycorrhizal fungi and bacteria complex. I used some slight training by bending the stems. This time I got just a bit shy of 400g under this 400W HPS in 12 weeks starting from seed. Nearly 100g per plant in a 2 liter container!

While applying this method, I noticed the inflorescences had a higher calyx to leaf ratio than you'd normally see. There was very little leaf production overall.

What are your thoughts and take on this?

Dominique

_____

Growing from seed to flower under a regimen of 12 hours is a viable cultivation technique and your experiments were typical of the success people have with it.

One way to figure the success of the garden would be to look at the yield through the lens of watts per gram.

Let's say that two gardens had the same yield and used the same number of watts per day but one took 8 weeks from seed (or clone) and the other took 10 weeks. Obviously the 8-week garden was the bigger yielder. Here's a formula to figure it. Yield divided by total watts, that is, yield divided by bulb wattage x number of hours daily x number of days. Here it is applied to the 8-week cycle 400 (grams)~.4 kilowatts (kw) x 12 x 56= 268kw. 400~268=1.49 g per watt. The 10-week cycle light formula: .4 x 12 x 70=336 kw. 400(g)~336= 1.19 grams per watt.

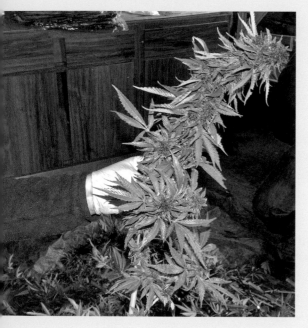

FINISHING TEMPERATURE

What should the temperature and humidity be for the last two weeks of flowering?

Marijuana grows fastest when the leaves at the top of

the canopy have a surface temperature of about -2.22 to -1.110. So the fastest growth and ripening will proceed in this range.

However, this is not the only consideration. The terpenes, the odor molecules that give varieties of marijuana their "personality", are oils that are volatile at relatively low temperatures. That's why marijuana odors waft through the air on warm days. The smallest molecules evaporate when the temperature range is -6.11 to -3.33 degrees. So by lowering the temperature the terpene content is increased but at the cost of slower ripening.

One compromise would be to lower the temperature for just the last 5 days.

Boveda. | The original terpene shield.™

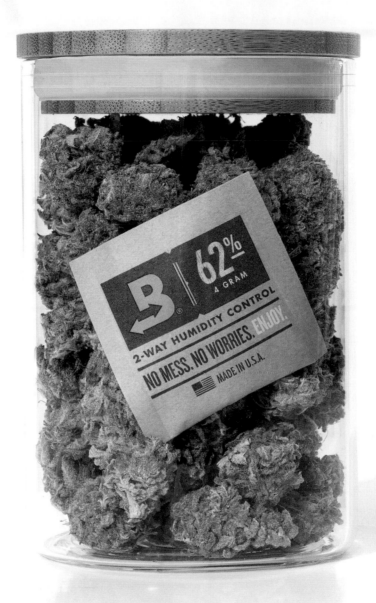

Boveda is the Original Terpene Shield™ that adds or removes pure water vapor to stored cannabis to:
- Create a monolayer of moisture that naturally coats trichomes
- Shield terpenes, so they don't evaporate
- Protect flower from over drying and mold growth

Maintains 58% or 62% RH levels, using nature's original preserver, salt.

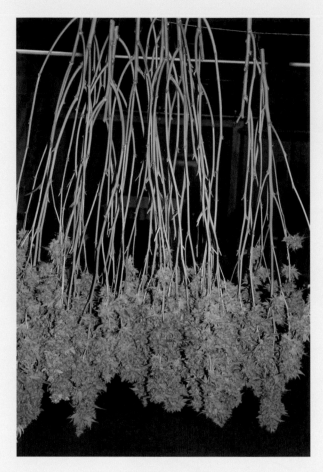

PARTIAL HARVEST

The top buds of my plants are mature and I'm about to harvest. However, the buds a little lower than the top of the canopy are not ready. Can I cut the tops and let the rest of the flowers go for another week or two? What disadvantages are there if any?

Yes. You can harvest just the mature portions of the buds that usually extend from the top of the canopy down four to six inches. Below that point, buds are sometime immature. These flowers exhibit new growth, fresh or undried stigmas, and trichomes with crowns that are not completely filled with resins.

When the mature portions are removed, the plant focuses its energy on these flowers, providing them with more sugars used for development and ripening as they begin to receive more intense, unshaded lighting. The flowers won't grow much more but they will mature and the trichomes will fill with resins.

LATE HARVEST FOR SALVE MAKING

I am growing a one to one CBD–THC strain for the purpose of making a salve. I'm looking for body pain relief more so than a head high. what effect would letting the trichomes turn amber or beyond have?

The trichomes' change of color from clear to amber or cloudy white is an indication of the transformation of THC to CBN. CBN is much less psychoactive than THC but provides pain relief and is anti-inflammatory. It would be a good ingredient to include in salves. Harvesting late, after some of the glands have changed color, is a good way to assure their presence.

CURING IN JARS

I am in the process of curing my buds in storage jars. I've been opening and checking on them daily and am also using humidipaks to keep the humidity in the jars as close to 60% as possible. However, I have to leave town for a few weeks and have no one to continue the process. Will they survive being sealed with the humidipaks in the whole time or should I look for someone to come care for my buds while I am gone?

———————————

Once the humidity packs are saturated they cannot collect more moisture and the relative humidity (RH) in the jars will soar. The moist air is a perfect environment for bacteria to thrive. The solution is to dump the jars and instead make a little enclosed space to maintain steady RH of 60%. Depending on the environment, you will probably either require a humidifier or dehumidifier that is regulated using a sensor. Dehumidifiers increase the temperature so an air conditioner may also be required to maintain a temperature of 700.

By keeping the buds at 50-60% humidity they will retain about 12% moisture, which is perfect for smoking.

FINISHING PRODUCTS

In your book, Marijuana Harvest, you talk about finishing products and their ingredients. I have been growing for about 7 years (2) rooms using a popular brand's planting mix and fertilizers products with success. Now I'm wondering if I'm missing out, just sticking to one line?

———————————

If you are curious about some of

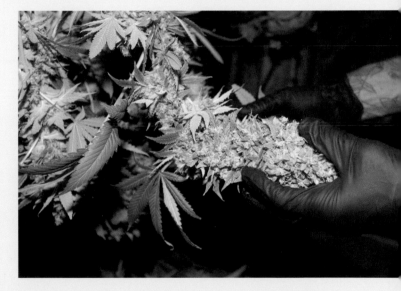

the bud enhancers and finishing products mentioned in Marijuana Harvest you owe it to yourself to experiment with them. Set aside a separate space or separate irrigation system to test them against your standard fertilizers and enhancers and make sure to keep all other conditions the same. Please report back.

The manufacturers of these products depend on repeat sales. If they don't work, who will buy them a second time?

Chapter 18

Garden Fever

Covers:
- Exploring different hydroponic methods
- Simple light deprivation methods to speed up ripening

Growing marijuana is habit-forming, if not addictive. I know cultivators who have given up using marijuana but still grow it. I know from personal experience that the first is true: growing is definitely habit forming. However, I have not given up using it.

In June, a friend brought over four "Ed Rosenthal Super Bud" single stems that were just going into their 2nd week of flowering. Then another friend came with some of their excess OG and OG crosses. A third brought some local varieties. It would have been heartless to turn these orphans away, so I decided to give them a home in my greenhouse.

I set up a 2'x8' tray for the adoptees. Both feed from the same reservoir. One group of plants is in 6" containers on a wick system in planting mix with supplemental drip sits on a platform above the tray with wicks trailing into the tray. The other group is in 2.5 quart containers, each made from two Dollar Store plastic colanders. The bottom third of each sits in water so the plant's roots can easily migrate into it.

ONE MONTH LATER

One month later, the plants there are doing fabulously. I have plants in two different systems drawing water from the same tray. The first uses clay pebbles. The 8" tall colanders are submerged 2" and above water 6". A pump constantly delivers a gentle stream of water that flows over the pebbles, creating a water/nutrient film. Large air spaces between the pebbles provide the roots with plenty of

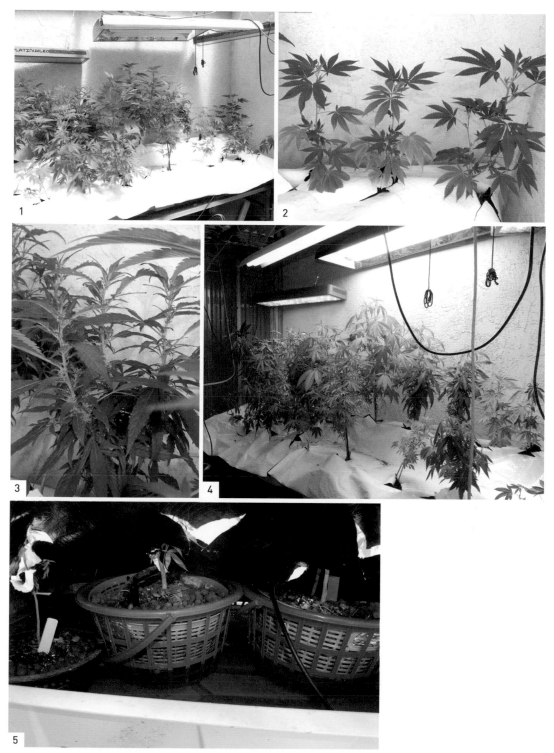

1. The greenhouse during the day. The plants get about 5 hours of direct sunlight, and an additional 5 hours of indirect bright light.   **2.** Plants have acclimated to their new environment and are growing quickly.
3. The main stem was topped 10 days before flowering. 3 branches grew in its place.
4. Greenhouse by lights. This photo, taken at night shows how the plants are lit using fluorescent and LED lights. They are on 7-10AM and 4-8PM to supplement natural light.   **5.** The hydro system: Colander containers hold the hydrcorn but allow a free flow of water. Notice that roots are beginning to grow into the reservoir.

air. The other group of plants uses a planting mix and is irrigated using a wick system. Nylon rope hangs from holes in the bottom of the containers into the tray. Water is drawn up to the container as it used by the plant by capillary action, the same way a tissue draws water. In addition the container receives about a 8 ounces of water 3 times daily using a timer to regulate a small submersible pump.

The plants have grown extremely tall – they're approaching the greenhouse's 9' ceiling. Looking at the situation, I realized the tray was sitting on a table and I'd need to remove it in order to provide the plants with additional room.

Friends helped me empty the tray of the plants, drain the water, remove the tray from the table, and then place it on a Styrofoam board to stop heat transfer with the greenhouse floor, and then reassemble the unit.

Then the tray was put back together. Later this month (July) the plants will be light-prepped for a mid September harvest.

SEASONAL TIP: GARDENING INTO FALL

It's still not too late to plant with seed or clones outdoors or in a greenhouse in areas where it stays warm through the end of October. In other areas plant in containers that can be moved outdoors on warm days and lit indoors on cool or rainy days. The plants will immediately start to flower as they grow and will be ready to harvest in 60-70 days.

It is August and, the plants in the greenhouse are doing very well. The top buds were again approaching the ceiling but I bent them or clipped them to avoid it and to encourage top growth of the strong side buds.

Almost all the plants were lollipopped. The small branches with tiny buds were removed, so that they would not thwart growth of the larger top buds. This opens up the space so there's less humidity and more light getting to the important buds and their supporting leaves. All of these plants are being grown hydroponically. The ones in the back are in planting mix and watered using a wick system supplemented by drip watering from the reservoir twice a day, supplying the plants with about 10 ounces of water daily. The plants in the front are planted in hydrocoral in eight 8" high plastic colanders sitting half submerged in water. These plants are also irrigated by a constant drip.

The plants are in their second to third week of flowering. In the next week I'm going to install blackout curtains to speed up flowering by allowing the plants only 11 hours of light daily. I hope to harvest in 6 weeks, at the end of September.

The outdoor garden is in a 2'x4' hydroponic tray with 1.5 gallon containers filled with hydrocoral. They are sitting in the tray with a constant drip irrigation system. They get about 5 hours of direct sun and bright light the rest of the day. In addition, they receive light reflected from the white wall behind them. These plants are in the first stage of flowering. To speed up the flowering process I plan to start using light deprivation in the coming week, helping the plants to ripen by mid-September, while the days are sunny and warm, avoiding the iffy weather later in the season.

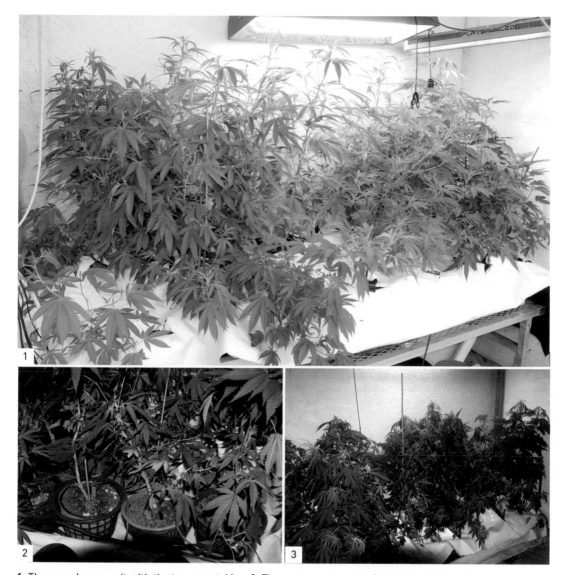

1. The greenhouse unit with the tray on a table.   **2.** The water systems are installed and tested.
3. The tray (now positioned lower) to allow more room for growth.

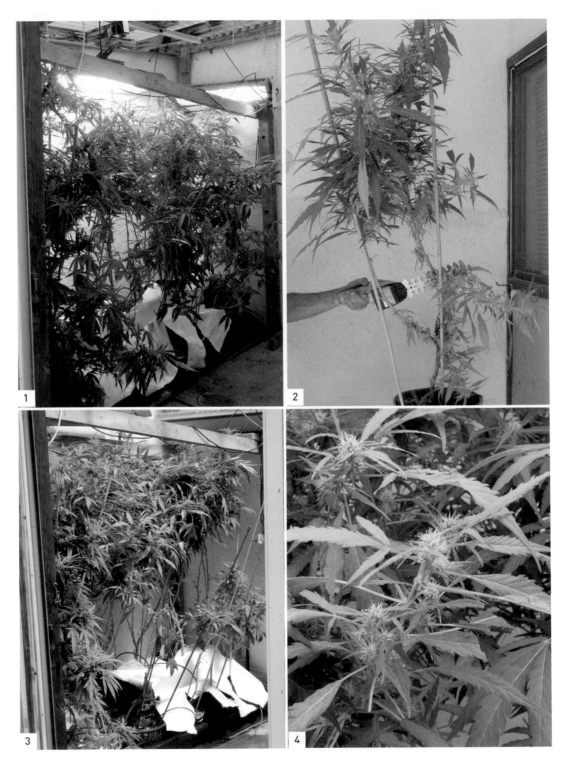

1. The plants in the greenhouse. Small lights turn on automatically early in the morning and then again in late afternoon to supplement the limited natural light. 2. Lollipopping a plant: removing the lower portions and smaller buds. 3. The greenhouse in direct sunlight with lolipopped plants. 4. Early budding on the ER Super-Bud plants, 2 to 3 weeks into flowering. 5. The outdoor system—plants are thriving and in the early stages of flowering.

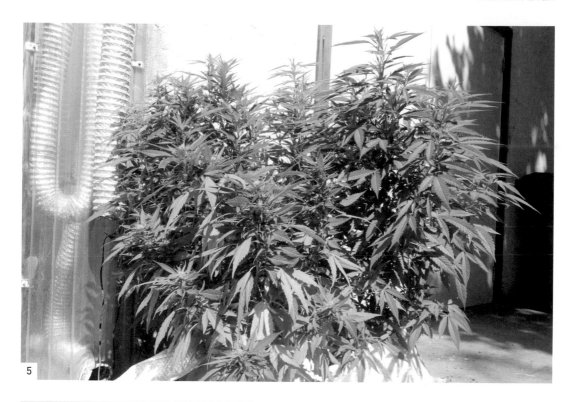

5

AUTUMN BUD

An easy way to grow some bud in autumn is to place plants in an unobstructed south-facing window. The sun is at an oblique angle, rather than high in the sky, so it will shine directly on the plants for a good part of the day.

Perhaps you or a friend have some plants that are ready to flower. If not, you may be able to purchase some "adolescents" from your local pot shop. They can be flowered immediately. Just put them at the window and don't turn on lights, even for a moment, during the evening (dark period). Fertilize with bloom formula. They will soon start to bud.

If you have only clones, use them. If you want them to grow a little before flowering, do interrupt the dark period with light several times each evening. Soon after you stop the nightly interruptions, the plants will begin to flower.

A SIMPLE LIGHT DEPRIVATION SYSTEM

It is now September10th, time to harvest the first plant from my garden, a small Purple Pineapple. The plant is small, no bigger than 2 feet, with a top bud and a few small side buds. It has been growing in a 10" wide colander container filled with Hydrocoral in the 2' x 8' reservoir hydro unit in my small greenhouse

The garden was started in mid-June. The plants all started light flowering immediately because the 10 hours of darkness they received at the shortest night of the year (June 22) was long enough to induce flowering. With no vegetative growth period, the plants put all of their energy into the re-

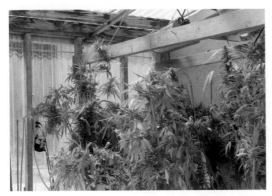

All the plants in the greenhouse are weeks way from ripening. Greenhouse receives natural light only through the roof and the front.

productive stage. This small plant, took the light more seriously than its buddies. Ripeness is the result.

The other plants in the greenhouse are in various stages of flowering. and will ripen by the end of the month. It's a good time for the plants to mature. In the San Francisco Bay coastal area, where the greenhouse is located, September is the warmest month of the year, with clear skies rather than the famous summer fog, and with little chance of rain.

Two systems are using the same reservoir in the greenhouse. The group in the back are planted in 2 to 4 gallon containers filled with a coir-based planting mix. The mix was enriched with plant meals, which release nutrients over several months. Nylon wicks hang from the bottom holes into the reservoir. The wicks, made using 3/8" nylon rope, carry water up to the containers from the reservoir un-

underneath. They use "capillary action", just like a tissue drawing up water. It self-regulates water uptake as needed. This action continues up the planting mix, replacing moisture as it is used by the plant and environment.

The plants also receive about a pint of water from the top 4 times daily using a repeating

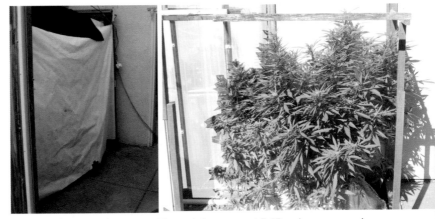

The greenhouse under wraps. The curtains go on at 5:45 and are removed shortly after sunset. The outdoor garden. These plants will ripen in early October. They will be moved into the greenhouse after those plants are harvested when there is room.

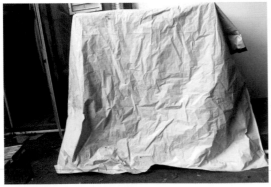

Outdoor garden under-cover.

timer that is set to run every 6 hours for 8 minutes.

The group in the front, use 10" colanders just like the one used to grow the plant harvested today. They sit in about 3" of nutrient water and have a constant flow of it pumped through the hydro-pebbles.

Water is pumped through the main line to the spaghetti irrigation lines directly to the top

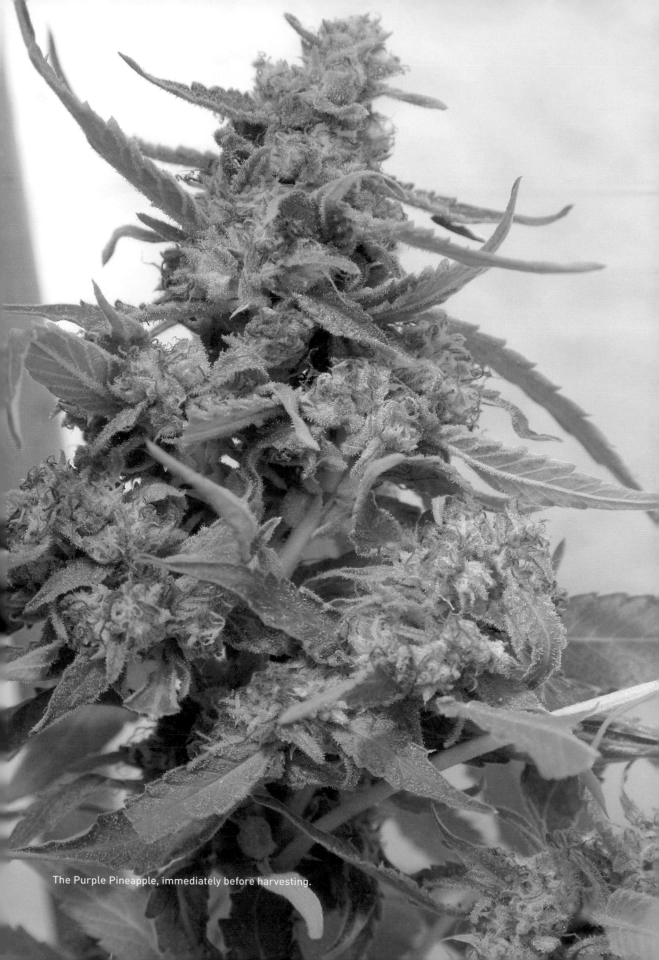

The Purple Pineapple, immediately before harvesting.

of the containers without the use of regulating emitters.

The third group consists of 5 plants in 2 gallon containers in a 2' x 4' try filled with planting mix. The tray was placed against the white wall that gets 6-5 hours of direct sunlight daily. One of these plants will also ripen and be harvested in 10 days. The other will take two weeks longer.

Cannabis is induced to flower by when the dark period reaches a critical level, which varies by variety. However, maturity can be hastened by increasing the dark period, signaling to the plant to stop flower growth and start ripening.

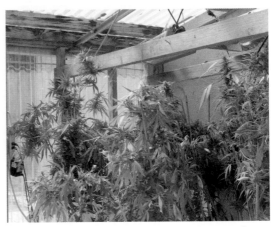

The greenhouse before the plants were harvested.

I decided to use this technique starting around August 20th to make sure the plants ripened a little early, in September under clear skies, rather than in October, when there is always a chance of weather problems.

To do this I devised simple light deprivation curtains that were placed over the gardens 11 hours after dawn, at about 5:45, rather than sunset at 7:25, blacking out the garden an hour and 40 minutes early. The difference in darkness was greater earlier in the cover-up, because the days were longer.

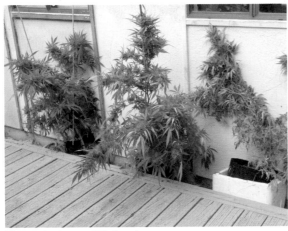

Three plants are still ripening.

HARVEST IS HERE!

The garden was in harvest mode for a month. The first plants to ripen were the Purple Pineapple. Then the Gelatos, both in the greenhouse and outdoors. The ER Superbuds, which were forced to flower barely out of clonehood, followed about a week later. These plants grew no branches, just a straight stem surrounded by buds.

There were also a couple of sativas that grew well vegetatively but never really budded out. The light wasn't bright enough for them. They were a waste in this garden- They took up space but were not worth harvesting. It was only in mid-season that I learned they were not clones but seedlings from an untested cross. Oh well.

Only two plants in the greenhouse and three outdoors were left. They need another 10 days to finish and luckily the forecast for the next week was for sunny and partly cloudy weather with highs in the 70's, perfect weather for plant ripening.

The position of the sun has changed with the season, placing it lower on the horizon. It casts more shade than direct light on the yard. I moved all of the plants to the sunniest section of the garden, outdoors. The plants were close to a white wall that reflected light back to them. This increased the total light they receive including UVb, which is blocked by plastic.

Meanwhile, the harvested plants were in various stages of drying/curing. When they were cut they were hung, unmanicured. The drying area has a bit of ventilation and a temperature that stays in the 60's and a humidity that remains in the 50 percent range. This is a great temperature/humidity combo for a slow dry/cure.

The first plants were smokeable dry and have been manicured. They have been placed in a jar with a humidity pack to keep them fresh.

So far I have manicured and smoked only the Purple Pineapple and the Gelato. The Gelato developed small dense buds a fruity odor. The smoke expands a bit and the first part of the high comes on quickly, then envelopes you with its rhythm. It's a good bud to socialize with.

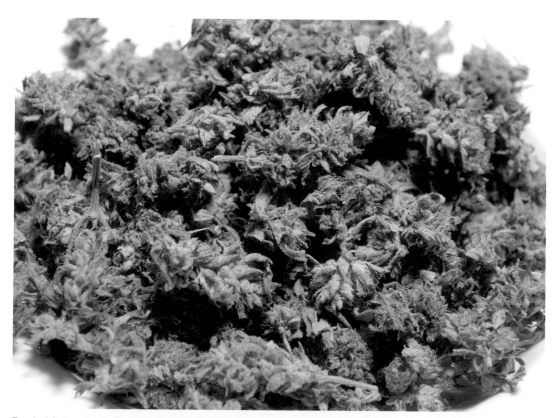

Bowl of Gelato buds. They would have been even tighter if they had more light.

Chapter 19

Ketama: Morocco's Cannabis Paradise

Covers:
- Traditional use of tight planting for greater yield

Close your eyes and imagine a land where almost every bit of arable space is planted with high-THC cannabis. If you opened them in the province of Ketama, in northern Morocco, that would be reality.

My partner, Jane, and I took a 3.5-hour flight from Amsterdam to Marrakesh, hung out there for a few days, then hired a car and driver for the 5-hour ride across the countryside to the Blue City, Chefchaouen, which flourishes on both domestic and international tourism. We saw no sign of cannabis in the two cities and rambling through the countryside. No paraphernalia in shops, no one using it, and certainly none in the fields.

That scene changed as soon as we crossed the border into the province of Ketama. It's in the Rif Mountains, which have a pattern of steep hills, protected valleys, and broad slopes. Its inhabitants are Berbers, people who have lived there for thousands of years and have their own culture, distinct from the rest of Morocco. And the only source of income is cannabis.

Before we set out, a friend arranged for us to meet a grower who lived fifteen minutes from the town center. He's newly married and lives with his wife in his family's house. His parents and his married brother and sister-in-law with two children also lived there.

The house is built around an inner courtyard. During the summer, much of the family daily routine takes place there. These activities include washing clothes, child rearing, and preparing food.

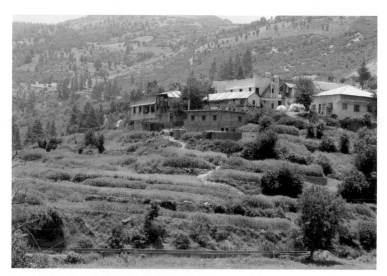

View of the area from the top of the mountain. The land is flat towards the town center and then the slope increases into steep mountains. Every arable space is used. More was created using terracing.

Women rarely leave the house except to work in the fields and for social events such as weddings, funerals, and some religious ceremonies. In town it's a man's world. The men do the shopping, spend time in diners and restaurants, and socialize in cafés.

We were ushered into a small room for guests, where we slept and were served meals. Our host showed us three bags of kief made from last year's crop—each a different variety. Hash making has improved tremendously over the thirty years since I first toured Morocco. When I first visited, I couldn't get high off the hash. Rachid's product was very satisfying.

Jane was treated with respect in her interactions with our host, Rachid, and in town. My interpretation of the situation is that she was treated as an "honorary male." While it would have been unusual and perhaps a little disruptive for a local woman to eat in a restaurant with her husband, diners were accustomed to seeing Western women. Jane was the only woman in the restaurants.

Rachid took us around his farm, which consisted of fields ranging from fairly flat to moderately steep slopes. Marijuana was planted everywhere. Of course, it did better on the flat land, which had more nutrients than on the slopes, where nutrients wash downhill with every rain. In some patches the leaves were yellowed. Adding nitrogen would have been an easy way to boost the vitality of these plants.

Our host gave us full access to his acreage and the surrounding farms. We continued along a dirt road that crossed fields on either side, and ran into a gaggle of kids tended by two teenage girls. Everyone wanted photos with us, and one of the older girls removed my sunglasses to take a selfie wearing them. These kids seemed to have a different set of expectations than their parents might have.

We spent one night with our hosts, but the space wasn't very comfortable, and

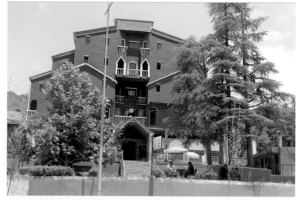

The Shotwa Hotel. Ketama's grandest. Our room cost about $20 a night. Hot water is available only on the first floor. The glory has faded but the bed was comfortable. No TV or AC.

because of its isolation we spent a lot of time waiting for Rachid while he was out and about on business.

Before he drove us back to town, he took us up the mountain. At the very top, the land was leveled flat and his cousin was building a large house there. The geography was plainly visible. These young mountains pushed up steep and jagged with a valley separating the peaks. Doing a 360, I could see that every section of land that could support a crop was planted in cannabis. It reminded me of Van Gogh's paintings of farms and fields. Differing techniques and the varieties being planted resulted in a patchwork of green and tan shades delineating each farmer's holdings.

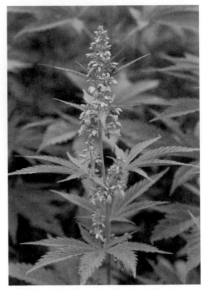

Male flowers. It's the first week of July and all the male plants are flowering. Even in midsummer the plants receive more than 10 hours of darkness, inducing them to flower.

Farmers here were still growing using the traditional technique of placing plants close together to produce a single bud. Done properly and supported by nutrients, this can be an efficient technique for commercial production because it would save the time and energy spent keeping plants in a vegetative state. Most of the farmers don't understand that a pollinated female plant will not produce a resinous bud. It would be better if they pulled the male plants so that the female plants' energy went into producing bud rather than seed.

There weren't many tourists in town, probably because it wasn't hash-buying season. In fact, there were so few guests at the Shotwa Hotel that we were assured of a "superior room." The room cost about twenty dollars; it was large and clean but didn't come with hot water. This structure, built when ski tourism was a major industry in the region, is a faded beauty.

The hotel was about 1,000 feet from city center, sitting on a rise. The climb from the street to reservation desk was about forty-two steps, then more to the room, not convenient for travelers lugging gear.

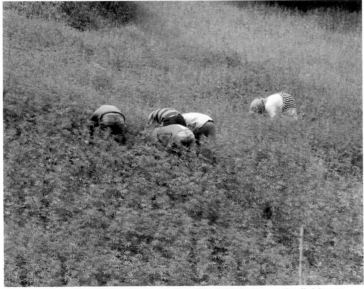

Workers removing males. It's an impossible task because the fields are so vast. Even if they were all removed, pollen from other fields would pollinate the females.

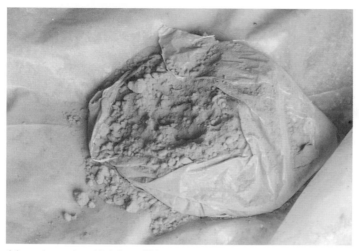

A bag of premium kief that will be pressed into hash. Years ago the hash was very weak. Interbreeding with modern varieties has increased its potency to acceptable levels.

Good exercise, though, to get in shape for some casual hiking on steep trails.

From the hotel window we had a view of the road and a construction site where I never saw any work being done. Beyond that, there were dirt banks denoting where a seasonal stream gushes into the spring and then the cannabis fields.

We were in a valley. The land was flat, and the plants were well cultivated and very healthy. I was looking at twenty-five acres right outside the hotel window. It was hilly at the back of the hotel, but parts of the slope had been terraced to make space for more cultivation.

We walked into town, then took a path to the nearby fields, passing a few people who smiled or greeted us as I was taking pictures. The fields were well cared for, resulting in some of the healthiest and most vigorous plants seen so far. Here, I noticed that several women did have the job of pulling out the male plants.

We left Ketama shortly after we took photos and traveled to Fez by car. It's a long journey because of the road winding its way through the mountains. The entire area, everywhere we could see, was planted with weed. It only stopped at the border of the district. At the official border the landscape abruptly changed into olive tree orchards, wheat, alfalfa, and other crops, but no cannabis was visible.

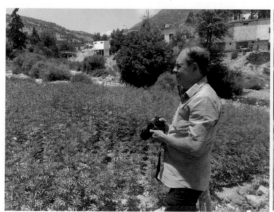
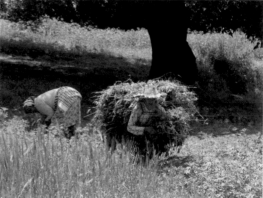

The author standing by a field with the city in the background.
After the males are picked they are bundled up and women carry them out of the field. They are fed to livestock.

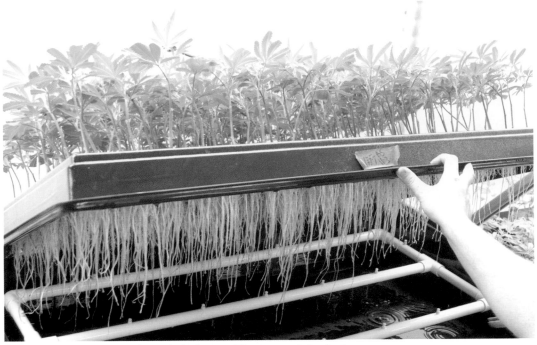

Aeroponically grown clones have six-inch roots. They are ready to plant.

Chapter 20

Colorado's Legal Cannabis Market:

Inside Kind Love's Marijuana Production Facility

Covers:
- Professional cloning techniques
- Air circulation techniques
- Tips for increasing efficiency at home or in a commercial garden

Medical marijuana has been permitted in Colorado since 2010. Then, in 2012 voters legalized its use, sales, and production. With legalization came increased demand and of course more production. Now, instead of having surreptitious grows of 10–20 lights, producers are using spaces that accommodate hundreds to thousands of lights.

While I was in Colorado recently I had the opportunity to visit Kind Love's marijuana production facility. I was immediately impressed by the hygienic nature of the facility. There was no dirt, no extraneous matter. Nothing was out of place, nothing was laying around, and no garbage was to be seen.

ABOUT THE GROW SPACE:

Kind Love divides its grow space into rooms, each with 40 double ended air-cooled HPS lamps mounted on the ceiling, which is about 14 feet high. Although the lamps are further from the plants than in most grow rooms, little light is lost because almost all of it shines directly on the canopy. The light hitting the walls is reflected back into the garden area.

All of the equipment used to maintain each room's environment is located outside the room so there is no reason to go into growing areas for adjustments or repair. Each room is individually controlled as far as light regimen, temperature, humidity, and CO_2.

THE GROWING PROCESS:

The growing process starts when clones are taken from mother plants, which are about 5 feet tall and are kept active for six to eight months. The clones are rooted in aeroponic cloning systems. When the roots hang down about six inches the clones are rooted in one-gallon containers in a mix consisting of coir fiber and perlite. The non-nutritive medium is fertilized using Botanicare products in a drip to drain system.

After two weeks most of the varieties are repotted into three-gallon containers, but kept growing vegetatively for another week. A few varieties are kept in vegetative for longer periods because they are slower growers.. During the entire vegetative process the plants are grown under fluorescent lights. The lights are kept on for 18 hours a day.

After one to two week in their larger containers, all varieties, are forced to flower by changing the light regimen to12 hours. The containers are placed on 2½-foot spacing. Each flowering room contains several compatible varieties.

Colorado law calls for 70 percent of the product sold at each shop to be produced at a dedicated facility. So, all of the bud produced at the facility is sold at Kind Love's dispensary in Denver.

TECHNIQUE AND EFFICIENCY:

Although the facility is well run and the plants are healthy and productive, there are some inefficiencies in the system and its caretaking regimen.

Whether you are growing a small garden or a large facility the plants respond the same way to environmental conditions and care. What changes is the methods that you use to provide that environment.

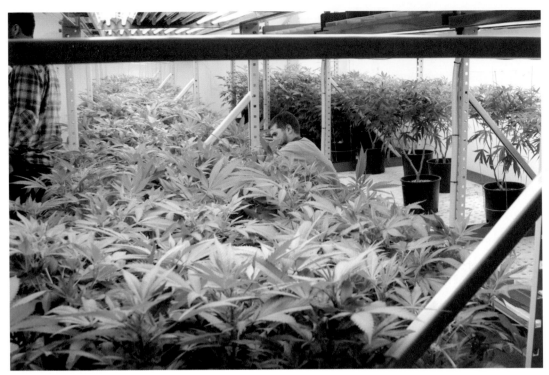

Vegetative plants grown under fluorescents (in foreground) are ready for repotting. Mother plants can be seen in background.

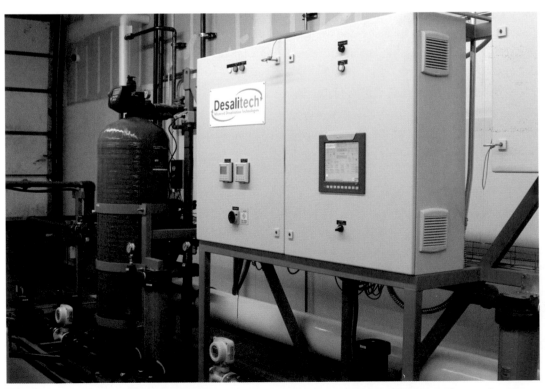

All room controls, such as temperature/humidity, CO_2, and water, are kept outside the garden space for easy access.

1. If the plants were forced to flower when they were smaller they would spend less time in the vegetative state, speeding up rotation by 2 weeks, reducing the cycle from 11-14 to 9-10 weeks, an average of a 24% time reduction. There are also labor savings from reduced transplanting and pruning. Additional costs would come from a larger pool of mothers to take clones and additional production of clones.

2. If you are subject to plant counts the present regimen would be a good one to follow. By buying clones if available, you shortcut the plant's journey to ripeness by two to three weeks, In 3 weeks the plant is ready to flower. With each plant using about 2 ½ foot square, the plants will fit into a 5' x 5' space.

3. Plants are being grown under fluorescents that produce only two-thirds of the light of HPS lamps. LED fixtures can be used to replace them.

4. Some of the plants are hand-watered. This wastes time and is not as effective as automated systems.

5. Government regulations specify that if a space has a single infection, all the plants in the room must be dumped. For this reason there is an incentive to keep each room small. With more realistic regulations there would be an incentive to create large spaces, which are more economical to maintain.

6. During my visit it wasn't clear to me how are the pots filled with soil. Ideally, they grower should be using automated potting equipment.

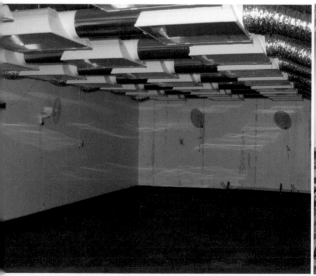

The facility is still being developed. This room is being set up.

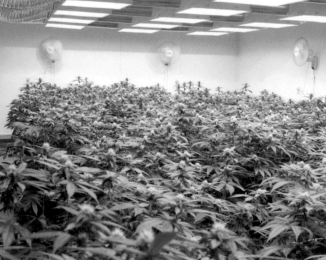

These indica hybrids are a month from ripening.

Ask Ed   COMMON LIGHTING QUESTIONS

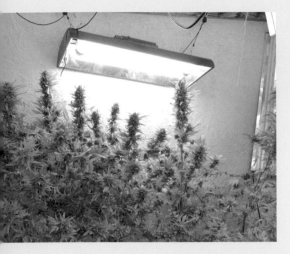

DISTANCE FROM LIGHT

I have a 600w HPS light. When the plants were 4" tall I moved the light from a meter above them to 50 cm. Now the plant leaves are deformed and shriveled, but they are growing again and the leaves are flattening out.

What distance would you keep the lights in vegetative and flowering?

Outdoors, marijuana grows in full sun, even at low latitudes, where the light is very intense. These plants grow long "palisade" cells to modify the intensity before it reaches the center of the leaf. Leaves that have been grown under less intense light and then are placed under stronger light have not modified their morphology and can suffer light damage. When you reduced the distance by half, light intensity quadrupled. This may be a reason why the leaves were injured. The new leaves, which are growing under the more intense light, are adapting their structure for the stronger light and will not suffer.

When plants are moved outdoors in early summer, the strong UV light, which causes sunburn in humans, can injure the unprepared leaves. They should be protected until they have adjusted by first placing them in light shade, spraying an anti-transpirant such as Wilt-Pruf®, or placing a thin cloth such as lace over the plants so the plants don't get the light's full intensity. After a few days the old leaves will adjust a bit and the plants can receive stronger light. Another solution is to move the plants on cloudy, overcast days.

The closest distance that you can place lights to plants is not a factor of the light intensity, but of the heat and infrared light emitted by the reflector. While reflectors without a glass plate emit so much heat that they must be placed a meter or more from the canopy, reflectors with glass plates that are air-cooled can get much closer.

The best way to determine the minimum distance between light and plants can be determined using a surface temperature thermometer, which uses an optical beam aimed at the leaf canopy. The leaf temperature should not go higher than 78°F. With CO_2 enhanced air the plants grow well at temperatures up to 85°F or even slightly higher. Adjust the room temperature, light height, and air circulation to target these temperatures.

CONSTANT GREEN LIGHT

I left a green light on at night in the final week of flowering. What effect will this have on the plants?

Marijuana is a short-day plant, which means that its flowering cycle is based on the number of hours of uninterrupted darkness it receives. It measures light and darkness based on red and far-red light and, to a much lesser effect, based on blue light.

Short-day plants are not affected by green light in regard to the flowering cycle, so it is safe to leave a green light on during the flowering period. Both LED and fluorescent green lights do not emit red light so they are excellent sources of green light.

LIGHT INTENSITY

I use 16 1000-watt HPS lamps with Adjust-A-Wings reflectors. I like them because their parabolic shape spreads the light more evenly over the entire garden, which eliminates shadows and ultimately increases overall yield. Unfortunately, it's difficult to use these types of reflectors and get higher than 54,000 lumens per square meter at the canopy without heat issues, especially when multiple strains are being grown and the canopy becomes less uniform.

My question: If my priority is to grow the highest-quality product instead of maximizing yield, should I use focused reflectors instead?

Most cannabis plants grow very well and produce high yields under 54,000 lumens per square meter. The plants that are most likely to improve with increased light are sativas and sativa–indica hybrids.

The problem with the parabolic lights you are using in terms of increasing light intensity is that the reflectors have a big footprint and cannot be placed close to each other.

One solution to your problem of trying to increase light intensity is to use HO or VHO fluorescent lamps in addition to the lamps that are already installed. These 120cm tubes vary between about 50–100 watts. High-watt compact fluorescent lamps are also available. All these tubes are fairly efficient and can be mounted between or under the HPS lights.

LED DISTANCE FROM CANOPY TOP

I recently purchased two 300-watt LED lamps in 9-band spectrum to replace my two HPS energy guzzlers.

The lights emit no heat, which was the main factor for keeping those HPS and MH lamps 18 inches 45cm above the plants using air-cooled lights or 90cm without the bottom glass plate. What distance from the plants should the lights be placed?

Place the lights about 30cm above the top of the canopy. Since most LED fixtures contain multiple spectrums of bulbs, the distance allows the spectrums to spread more evenly over the canopy.

Chapter 22

Oakland Garden: Is This the Largest Urban Grow in the United States?

- Large scale container growing
- SOP (Standard Operating Procedure) for harvest

It wasn't long ago that the idea of growing an acre of marijuana was just a fantasy. But in 2016 California voters voted affirmatively on a partial legalization initiative.

Now we can see the short-term results. Commercial grows expanded from Mendocino type gardens typified by large plants, which each had a yield of 10-15 lbs. While staying within the plant limit, which usually ranged from 6 to 49 plants, growers were able to harvest relatively large crops. Indoors, a hundred light facility, with a canopy of 1500-2000 sq. feet was consider large.

Those are antiquated numbers now. Here in California the law allows outdoor farms of an acre or more. There are a number of outdoor farms in legal counties, but most of the large ones are in rural areas, where there is ample space to spread out.

However, in an urban area of California there was an acre plus lot that had just been cleared of derelict buildings. The soil was suspect. Before it was cleared abandoned cars and old machinery had been dumped there. However, the land was level enough to cover it with 20-gallon bags irrigated using a drip system.

The new owners were planning to construct a greenhouse on the land, but that was only in the

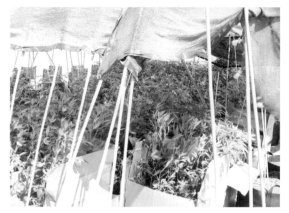

Plants were kept in the shade until they were transplanted.

planning stages. The space was not scheduled for improvement after the growing season was over. However it needed some modifications before it could be used. City water would have to be hooked up. That wasn't much of a problem. Before plants could enter a chain link fence marking the perimeter had to be made visually impenetrable.

Rather than buying filled bags the grower decided to buy bulk soil and have laborers fill the bags from a soil pile dumped in the middle of the space using shovels. As the bags were filled, they were set in place and then planted.

One the containers were in place the stakes and netting were installed. The stakes crossed each other and were tied. Then the netting was attached to the stakes. Finally, the branches were spread apart and attached to the netting using twist-ties. Unfortunately, the final garden design was not followed and the netting was set at an oblique angle to the sun. As a result portions of the plant that would have been sunlight were partially shaded. The correct angle would have been for the plants to face N/S , perpendicular to the sun. This becomes especially important in the fall, when the sun drops

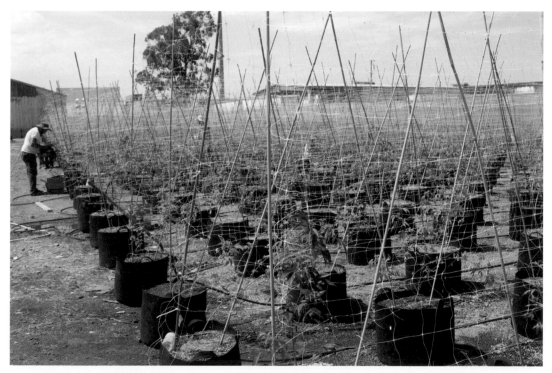

The stakes were tied together and then the netting was attached. Finally the branches were tied to the netting. No branches stuck out from the rows, much like the way wine grapes are trained.

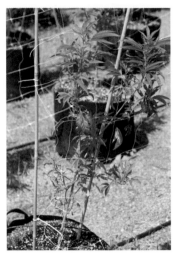

Twenty days after the first photo, plants have recovered and new growth is healthy.

in relationship to the horizon, casting longer shadows.

The cannabis plants had been growing under lights for several months but the intensity was low so the stems were somewhat stretched and the leaves were small. The six-inch containers were slightly rootbound. The situation wasn't critical and the roots would be able to grow into the new planting mix.

It turned out that the planting mix was not ripe so the plants were held back a little for the first two weeks by pH instability, causing unavailability for some of the micro-nutrients. Another problem that the plants faced was sunburn. The plants had been growing indoors under HPS lights, which emit no UV light. The old leaves got sunburn, just as a light skinned human not used too summer sun would.

In spite of all these problems, the plants adjusted to their new environment and the newest growth showed that the soil problems had been resolved.

*Once the plants were in place, the day length was already growing shorter and the longer night would induce the plants to flower. To prevent that, a person walked the rows twice each evening carrying an HPS lamp, which broke the dark cycle forcing the plants to reset their time count. This prevented them from flowering.**

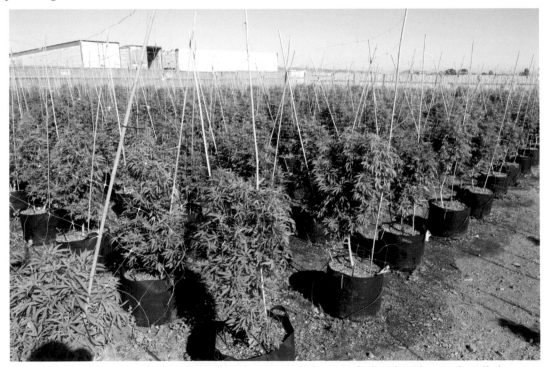

The field is about an acre and holds about 2800 20-gallon containers. Agricultural netting was installed on each row. The square are XXX" wide and the plastic is 8 feet high. It is held using an improvised "W" method of attached 8' long bamboo poles. Plant stem and branches are woven through the plastic so no tying is required.

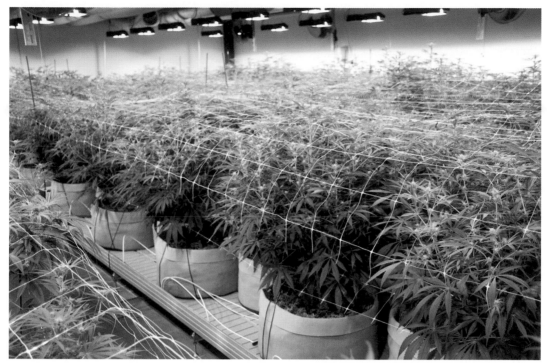

Commercial growers often use Smart Pots, the original fabric aeration container, to increase root mass and maximize yield. The container you use will affect plant growth. Aeration containers such as Smart Pots will help.

THE BUDS APPEAR!

Six weeks later, the plants had grown considerably and were allowed to flower. Normally these plants would have been tipped into flowering by the longer nights in mid-August. To keep the planters growing vegetatively, at first a caretaker slowly walked a 400-watt HPS lamp slowly down the rows each night near midnight. Later in the season HPS lights mounted on a rolling cart supplied dark-breaking light. Breaking the dark period halfway through the night resets the countdown so the plants never receive the 10-11 hours of uninterrupted darkness they require each night to start flowering.

Night lighting was stopped on Sept 7, so the plants were expected to ripen between the last week of October and the first week of November.

Several rows of plants were not treated with flashed light. They started flowering in mid-August and had another 4 or 5 weeks until ripening. They were considerably smaller than the treated plants. However they had tight premium buds that will definitely ripen before bad weather typically sets in.

- The next step was to prepare for harvesting and processing. We anticipated a minimum of about half a pound per plant, so preparations were made for processing. We planned to clip the buds off the plants while they were sill in the field and then hang them to dry. Everything was still in the planning stage because there were several options:
- Hang the whole plants. Process when dry.

- Hang the branches with buds to dry. Then de-stem the buds and manicure them using auto machines.
- Clip the plants and run them through debudder machine
- Clip the buds or use debudding equipment and manicure the buds using a roller machine. Then place them in trays to dry.
- Cut the buds from the plants in the field. Then slice the stems off the plants using power equipment. Then run the branches through de-budding machines to gather the leaves. Dry or freeze the leaves for further processing.

RAIN & PH ADJUSTMENTS

When the dark cycle lighting ended, the autumn dark period was long enough to immediately send the plants into flowering. All of their energy was devoted to reproduction and the plants were growing big buds in a vain search for pollen.

This variety of OG fills out late in the bloom period. The plants were now entering their 6th week of flower and they had about 2 weeks to go, so we expected to start cutting around November 1.

So far, nature had been good to this crop. We had a rainstorm in late September but it quickly dried with the help of a nice warm breeze. After that we had mainly clear, sunny skies with highs in the mid to high 70's, and nightly drops into the low 60's to high 50's. The humidity was high, ranging from 60-80%, but the constant salt air breeze coming off the Bay helps to keep fungi and molds from attacking the plants.

This was an outdoor crop so we were completely at the mercy of nature's vagaries. The forecast for the next two weeks was mostly sunny until the 29th, just before harvest, when cloudy weather and a slight chance of drizzle would hide the sun for three days. On Nov. 1, the scheduled harvest date, the sun began to peek through the clouds again.

If it rained, there was a good chance that the moisture and cool weather might promote germination of molds and fungi. To prevent this from happening, after the rain stopped we sprayed the plants with water pH'd to 8.5. The alkaline condition inhibits mold and fungi from germinating.

Our plan was to remove A buds and preserve them for sale as flower. They would be carefully dried and trimmed. The smaller buds and biomass wouldbe dried quickly using heat and very low humidity. Then they would be used for concentrates and extracts.

THE BUDS RIPEN!

The garden was ripe. As expected the buds were ripe on Nov. 1. However, there was a delay in preparing for it, and the crew was playing catch-up.

Every cultivator eventually learns that plants don't wait. No matter what your intentions, plants develop somewhat mechanistically; Inputs determine outcome/. Including timing.

The buds' ripening was a case in point. The light extension regime, interrupting the dark cycle by passing HPS lamps through the field several times a night, was ended on Sept 7., resulting in the plants switching to flowering from vegetative growth. At that point it was time to start preparing space to accommodate the plants that would be harvested. However, steps were taken only close

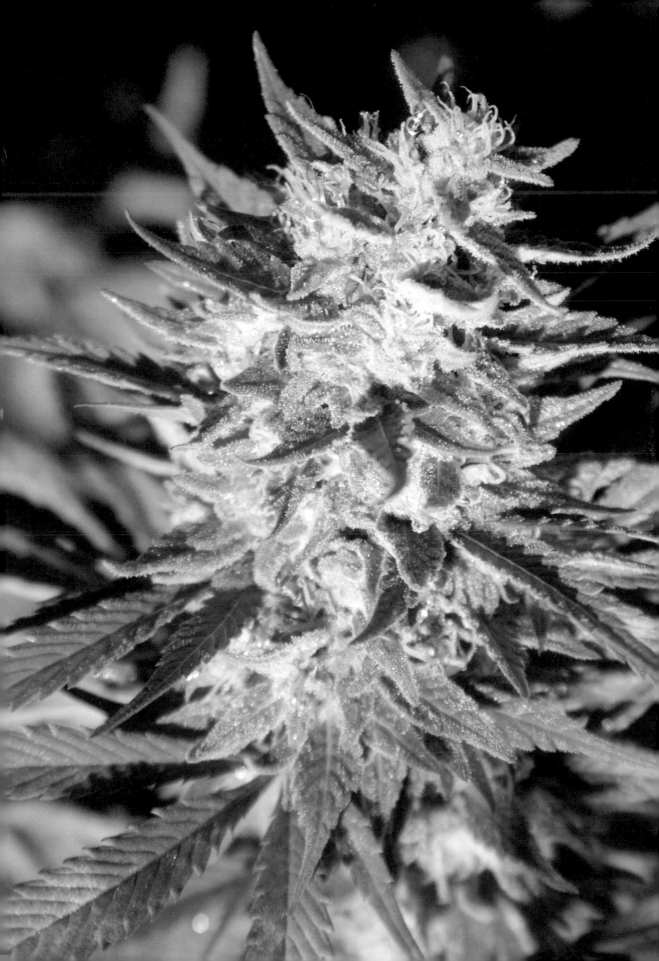

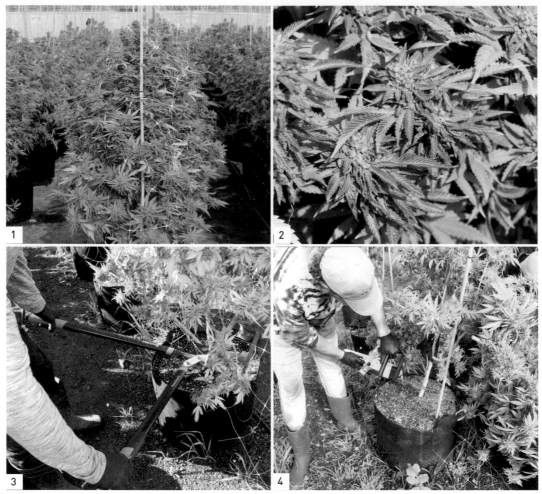

1. Mature plant is trellised so it has a width of less than 12 inches.   2. Close-up of buds. All but a few rows were OG Kush.   3. The plant is cut at the stem with a clipper.   4. A small chain saw makes the work faster and easier.

to ripening and have delayed harvest. The buds were ripe on Nov 1, as expected. However, the first drying lines were set up a week later. Then harvest began.

Today, Nov. 19, about 40% of the field has been harvested. We have been lucky as California suffered. Through October and early November California days featured clear bright sunshine with highs in the 70's and UV light ratings as high as 5.

These are the steps in the harvest process.

1. The plants are trellised using netting. It started with one layer of netting which the plant branches were woven into. Then, when the plants grew larger and had more branches, netting was wrapped over each side, so that there were three nets holding the plants in place.

   The outer nets had to be removed in order to clip the plants. At first crew members were cutting using small clippers. Later an electric mini hedge-trimmer was used to cut and remove the netting.

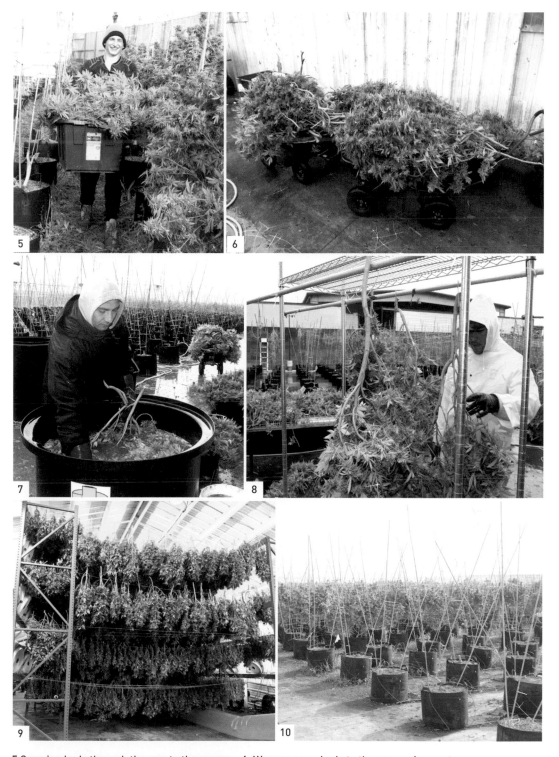

5 Carrying buds through the row to the wagon.   6. Wagons carry buds to the processing center.
7. The plants are dunked in a 1% hydrogen peroxide solution to protect against mold and bacteria.
8. They are hung to dry from the dip.   9. The drying rack is full. 10. Remaining plants in the field

2. Using a limb cutter at first, then later a small chain saw the plants are cut down and placed on small garden wagons.

3. The wagons are pulled to the processing area.

4. In the processing are the plants are dunked in 1% hydrogen peroxide solution and then hung on racks to dry outdoors. This prevents them from molding as they dry out.

5. The plants are cut into top and bottom sections and hung to dry.

6. The space is outfitted with a room dryer to keep the space warm enough for the plants to dry quickly. Fans re placed all around the drying area to support air circulation.

7. The plants dry in about a week and are placed in a separate areas to cure at 55% humidity for another two weeks.

8. After the plants have dried they will be sorted into A buds, smalls and concentrate material.

A RAPID HARVEST

Harvesting continued through November 27. There were several reasons for urgency in harvesting the plants. First, the buds were beginning to get overripe. Secondly, the weather, which

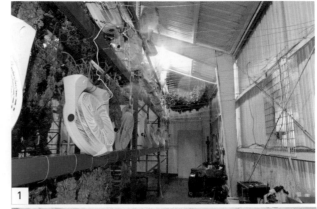

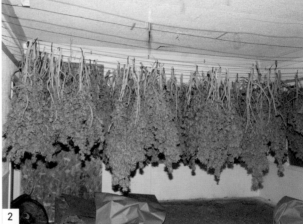

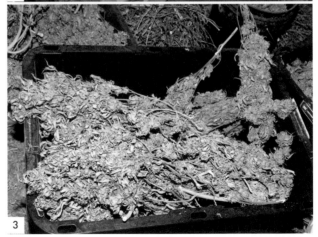

1. Fans keep the air circulating between the rows. 2. Some of the plants were hung. 3. Branches to be debudded.

had been amazingly sunny as a result of the drought in California, was about to turn. There were rainstorms on the 21st through the 23rd and then again on the 27th.

Except for Thanksgiving, harvesting continued through the 29th. The procedure was to cut the plants and place them in wagons to pull to the processing center. The plants were dunked in hydrogen peroxide solution to rinse off dust and dirt and kill spores and bacteria. Then they were hung to dry.

The drying frame was constructed of steel beams with 4 levels of wire hung across the area. Wire were spaced 3 feet apart to promote air circulation. The space was heated and dried using a blower powered by its own generator, which filled the room with warm air with an RH of less than 40%. The temperature was just under 800.. The perimeter of the drying area was surrounded with powerful fans that circulated air between the rows.

By the time the frame was filled with plants and bud, the plants that were hung earliest were dry and ready to be moved into the curing area. This consisted of a slightly cooler and more humid area. The plant branches were laid on craft paper only one cluster deep. Then another sheet of heavy craft paper was laid down and another layer of branches was placed on them. This was repeated five or six times.

Some plant tops were hung on wire along the walls increasing the capacity of the curing center.

After spending at least a week in the curing section the branches are bucked. This is accomplished in one of several ways. Either the plants are stripped by hand. Wearing heavy canvas gloves the branches are pulled

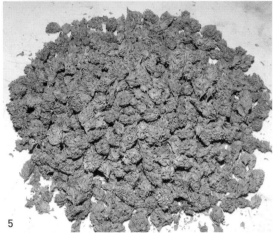

4. Workers de-budding the stems and branches 5. NBF (New Best Friend) Bud Pile Finished buds will soon be utilized using thermal papers or portable bud incinerators 6. The planting mix is open to the elements and gets rinsed out in the rain. This helps get it ready for the spring season.

through a mostly closed hand, stripping the plant. The stem is fed into a hole in the machine and it pulls t through, automatically removing the bud and other foliage. This really speeds up the process.

The buds are then being stored in cans. Until the buds are mostly dry they are kept uncapped. Only when they won't sweat when enclosed are the cannisters capped.

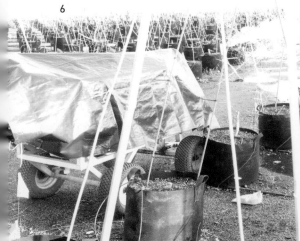
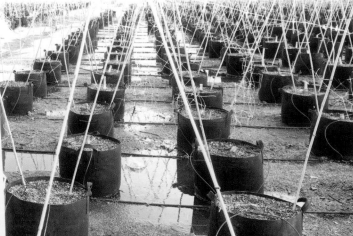

Chapter 23

Hashimals:
Enjoying the End Product

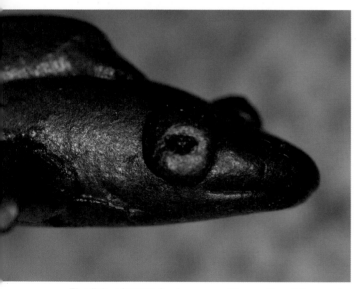

The fish, a bottom feeder, was set loose. Here it is searching for dried stigmas, the main portion of its diet.

As a result of genetic engineering, farmers all over North America are battling corporations such as Monsanto just for the right to continue to farm naturally. Consumers are facing Hobson's choices. Almost all soy grown in North America is genetically engineered. It makes it hard to eat healthy.

For this reason I was concerned when I heard that a medical marijuana provider was involved in a similar activity. Some friends mentioned that Oden was at a party and demonstrated how his recently created animals were able to do "tricks." Further, they had been developed using only plant genetics.

I called Oden, and he confirmed that he had indeed been acting as an "Intelligent Creator" and was planning on developing new creatures in the next few days. He invited me over to observe the delicate operations.

Upon entering the structure located in an old industrial section of San Francisco, I would never have suspected it to be a laboratory where new life forms are developed on a regular basis. It was designed to look like a loft apartment, and the specially designed equipment could have been mistaken for household items. I thought to myself that this was truly an ingenious way of keeping the research center discreet and under the radar.

Oden guided me to the lab bench cleverly disguised as a kitchen table. Getting to the point, I

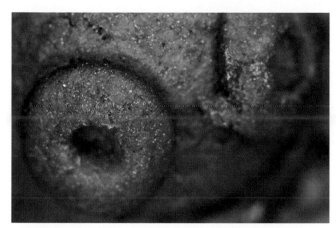

Two of the octopus' four eyes. Eye contact was good. So was eye-lung contact.

asked him if it was true that he had created animals using plant material. He said that he had. A wry smile, almost a smirk, escaped from the tiniest muscle in his lips and quickly spread to the other 25 muscles in his face.

He assured me that they were harmless, playful creatures. He was able to conceive them, he told me, but the creatures were not able to reproduce by themselves, so there has been no proliferation problem. "In fact," he mentioned, "I have given several of these as pets to friends, but all of them have disappeared into the vapor."

Then he said the words I wanted to hear, "Would you like to see my zoo?" I quickly affirmed my interest. Surprisingly, he opened a temperature controlled freezer unit. I thought, "The animals are kept in suspended animation at cold temperature, much like insects."

He must have read my mind because he said, "They only become pliable and lively when they reach room temperature." He gently removed the little golden objects from a zip-type plastic bag. They came tumbling out onto a soft towel.

I thought my hearing must be worse than I imagined. These aren't animals, they're hashimals. And of course they're made of plant material. What else would they be made of? Last time I looked, hash was a plant product.

Then he asked if I would like to watch him create a hashimal. "I sure would," I said.

Oden said that we should start with a freshly made piece of hash. He happened to have some on hand, so he was able to demonstrate his artistry. He started by taking an oval lump of golden water hash that he finished making just a few minutes earlier.

The hash was very soft and blond. It was wet to the touch and still contained a lot of water from the refining process. He placed it on a silk cloth, folded the cloth over it, and folded a towel over that. Then he pressed his palm on

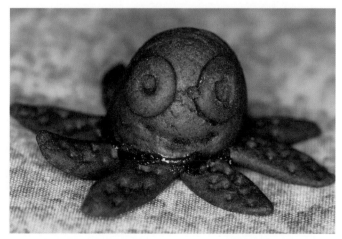

The wily octopus could not escape and it was dismembered to fit into the bowl.

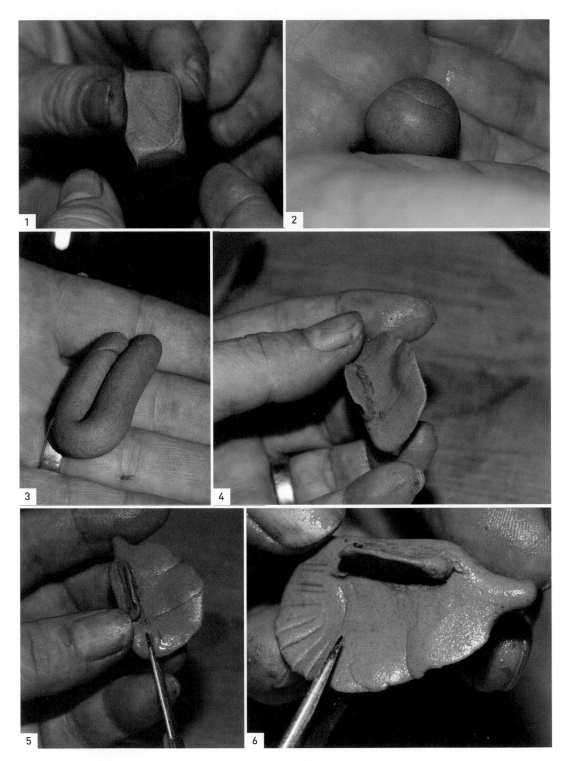

1. Steve, the Creator, started with a lump of clay.   2. He rolled it and it emerged as a ball.
3. Next the ball evolved into a worm like creature.   4. Deft hands flattened it and gave it symmetry.
5. Using specialized GE tools he caused a spine to evolve in the blink of a millennial's eye.
6. Using enhanced evolutionary tools the fish developed a dorsal fin and rays.

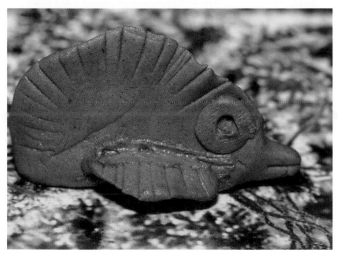

A black hasher was netted and smoked.

the towel, letting his weight act as a vise to press the water from the hash. The water passed through the silk cloth and was absorbed by the towel.

He used a knife to gently scrape the pressed material sticking to the silk. He lifted the scraping from the knife and pressed it into a solid piece. Then he used the sticky mass to collect hash still on the cloth. It was drier, but still very moist. He pressed it into a square and then started working on the sculpture.

He rolled it into a ball in the palms of his hands using a circular motion. As he rolled it, the surface sweated water. The surface became smooth and went from a matte finish to shiny. Then, instead of rolling his palms circularly, he moved them back and forth. The ball soon became a sweating log.

It looked a lot like he was working with clay. It was pliable and easy to mold and shape. Just like clay, some of it stuck to the skin and had to be scraped off.

Placing the fate of his creation in his hands, he folded the log over and shaped it into a rectangle. Then, using an unbent paper clip, he smoothed out the surface to an even layer. Next he started pressing the hash, making it thinner and giving the top a rounded shape. The extruded and pressed material miraculously formed side fins. The rounded back of the dorsal fin took shape.

The fish was evolving from a lump of "clay." Next, the fine detail showed the perfection of intelligent creation. Oden started to give his creation individuality. Using a pin, he developed a spinal cord with bones attached that held the fins in place. Picking up a few tiny pieces of primal matter, he rolled and flattened them and attached them to the unsighted creature, to give it at least a set of eyes. Voila! Another creature had evolved.

Here it was right before my eyes. Oden had taken plant material and, using the alchemy of modern science and technology, had made a golden sun-leaf fish. My fears were relieved because I knew that it had the likelihood of survival of a Chips-Ahoy® cookie at a kid's birthday party. No matter how many of these creatures come into being, they will be captured and, like salmon, smoked.

Oden has many of his creations in his exotic aquarium. There they bask in cool darkness and slowly lose their water and ripen. Little do they know that, as they grow older and lose weight, the day of their extinction grows near. Just as a human created these new forms, their existence will cease in a wisp of vapor and a little ash.

WILD ROOTS

My plants are in the flowering stage but the roots are coming out of the bottom of their pots. What do I do? Can I put a sponge in the tray to help keep them moist?

Using a moist, almost wet sponge is a great way to support the plants' roots. Sponges hold water but also have air spaces so the roots come in contact with Oxygen, which they require to stay healthy.

A couple of tips: Support the container on some sort of solid blocks so the sponge isn't squeezed. Make sure to keep the sponge moist at all times so the roots don't dry out.

SCROG NET HEIGHT

How much distance should there be between the base of the plant to a scrog net?

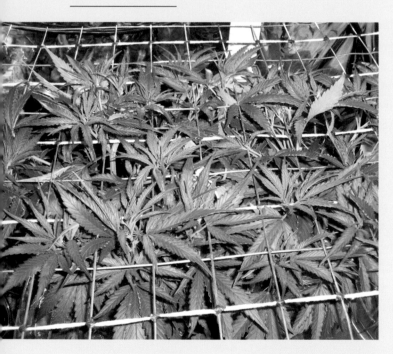

SCROG stands for Screen of Green-Plants are trained to grow horizontally on a screen. All the branches are kept at the same height so all the buds sites along all the branches are the same height from the light. They are more evenly illuminated than plants that are growing vertically. The plants are kept growing vegetatively until the canopy is mostly covered with vegetation.

To train the plants the tips are pruned at the fourth to sixth set of leaves. The plant grows two branches to replace the crown and some of the lower branches gain energy and are released from the effects of growth inhibiting auxin that was previously released by the top bud.

With no apical dominance all the branches will continue to grow and must be attached to screen or they will start vertical growth. By removing the growth tips the branches will divide, covering the screen faster and more completely.

The height of the screen varies depending on the technique you decide to use to divide the branches as well as the variety. Indicas can be SCROGED at as short a distance as 6-8 inches from the top of the container. Sativas stretch a bit and the SCROG unit is placed at a height of 15-20 inches.

MYSTERY PLANTS

I recently traveled to Jamaica where I was lucky enough to smoke some real quality buds. I kept and brought back 130 seeds which I germinated. I ended up with two very strong female plants. Is there any way of finding out their strains?

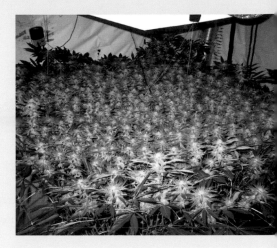

Jamaica had several landraces years ago, but cannabis connoisseurs and traders introduced modern European and American varieties to the island starting in the 1960's and continuing to the present. The landraces were obliterated because cultivators preferred the new varieties and cross-pollination.

Those seeds were probably derived from varieties or hybrids of varieties offered commercially. Still, there is a lot you can learn about the plants by their shape, size, growing habits, shape of leaves, color, bud shape and odor and the high. Getting a sense of all these factors will give you an idea of the varietal group they are from.

HOT ROOTS

I am having trouble keeping canopy and hydroponic roots at acceptable temps. The roots are too warm, way above 21°C. What should I do?

The problem with hot roots revolves around oxygen (O) in the water. The warmer the water the less oxygen it holds. Water at 690 holds considerably more O than at 720. There are two basic solutions to the problem.

Use a water chiller designed for aquariums. It will keep the water cool without contaminating it with unwanted metals such as copper. Units not made specifically for plants or aquariums should not be used because the plants risk contamination.

BETTER SEXING

I have 4 blueberry plants I started from seed about 2½ months ago. Last week I turned the lights to 12 and 12 to determine sex. The plants indicated within 3 days so I turned the light back to continuous so they would revert back to vegetative. Today I found one male sack about 4 or 5 branches down on one plant. This plant also is showing some white hairs. Should I get rid of it? And do you have any other tips to help me sex my plants?

The plant probably hermaphroditicized from the stress of the light changes. Nevertheless, it is not as stable as the other plants and should be discarded.

In the future sex your plants by taking a cutting from each one. Make sure that each is identified. Then place the cuttings in a space with lights on 8 and off 16 hours daily. Within a few days the cuttings will indicate. The clone's mother will have the same sex as the clone from which it was taken.

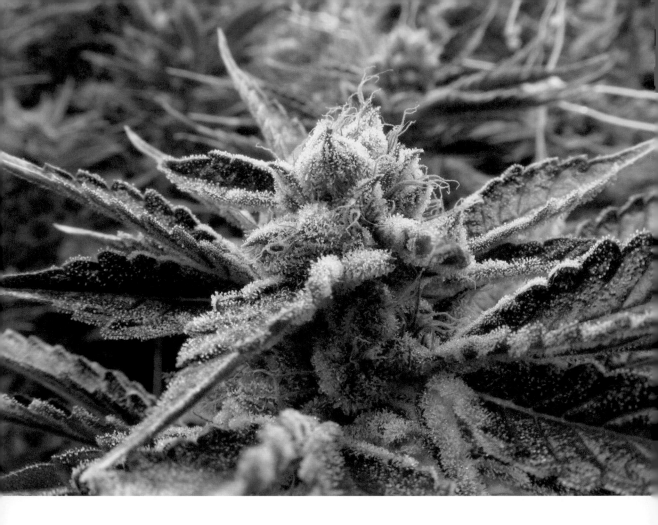

Sponsors

We would like to thank our sponsors, whose support and participation helped make this book possible.

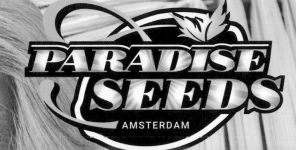

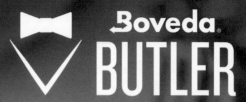

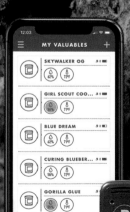
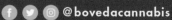

For growers who care about the yields *and* purity of their plants

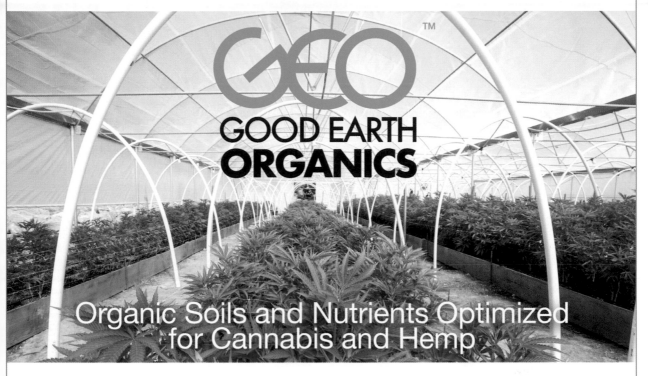

GEO™
GOOD EARTH
ORGANICS

Organic Soils and Nutrients Optimized for Cannabis and Hemp

Now more than ever it's important to know the plants we put into our bodies are grown without potentially harmful chemicals. **Good Earth Organics** soils and nutrients are **OMRI listed, Clean Green Certified,** and **approved for organic growing.** We carefully blend our products to ensure consistent performance and save you money because our soils can be reused for up to three harvests, reducing waste and expense. Our organic soils and nutrients work as a system, simplifying your grow and helping you boost plant performance and peace of mind knowing you are growing plants that are kinder to your body and to the planet.

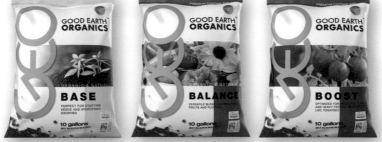

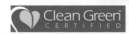

For more information on our products and for growing advice visit. the**good**earth**organics**.com
or call **833-GRO-PURE.** Available direct from our Oregon stores, on **amazon**, and in select retailers

HarvestMore

TRIM BIN SET

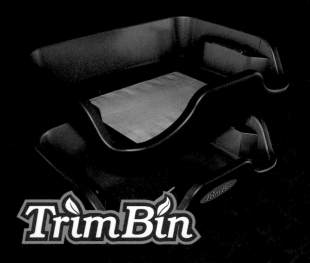

The Trim Bin by HarvestMore will turn any chair or surface into a comfortable work station. The high molded walls keeps your work contained and makes clean up a breeze. The Trim Bin is durable, portable, long lasting, and features an ergonomic design that makes trim work more enjoyable. The two part tray system allows for versatility and effcient use of space.

TRIM BIN FILTER

The Trim Bin FIlter has an additional sorting screen at its base that allows seperation of smaller materials into the attached collection bag. The Trim Bin Filter can also be nestled the the Trim Bin Set for additional sorting.

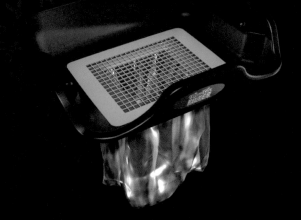

SCISSOR SCRUBBERS

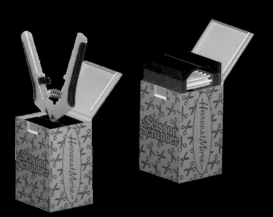

Get squeaky clean scissors in seconds with the Scissor Scrubbers. Just open the lid, remove the brushes and fill the container with your preferred cleaning solution, let your scissors soak, and use the rubber squeegies to clear off any excess solution.

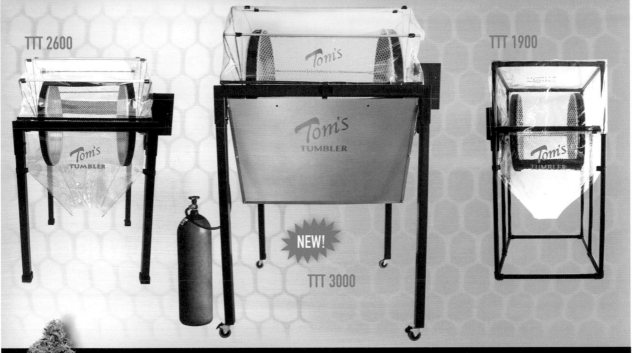
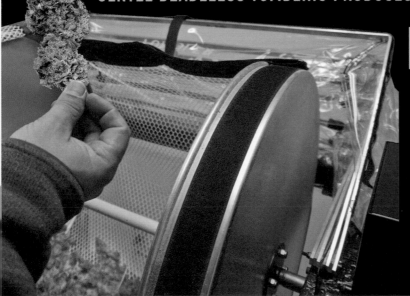
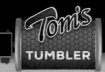

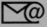

THE GREEN PAD CO₂ GENERATOR

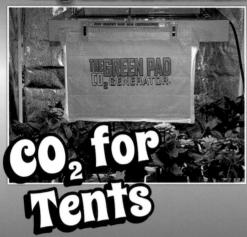

CO₂ for Tents

HUMIDITY ACTIVATED

THE GREEN PAD CO₂ GENERATOR JR.

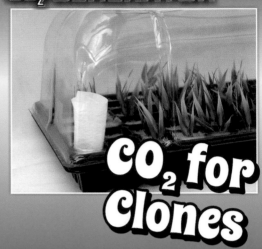

CO₂ for Clones

FASTER ROOTING!

THE GREEN PAD CO₂ GENERATOR GDP

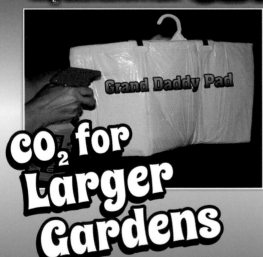

Grand Daddy Pad

CO₂ for Larger Gardens

HANG, SPRAY & WALK AWAY

Supplementing CO₂ in your indoor garden will give you bigger BUDS & heavier yields

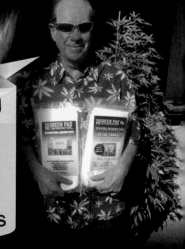

GreenPadCO2.com

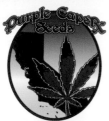
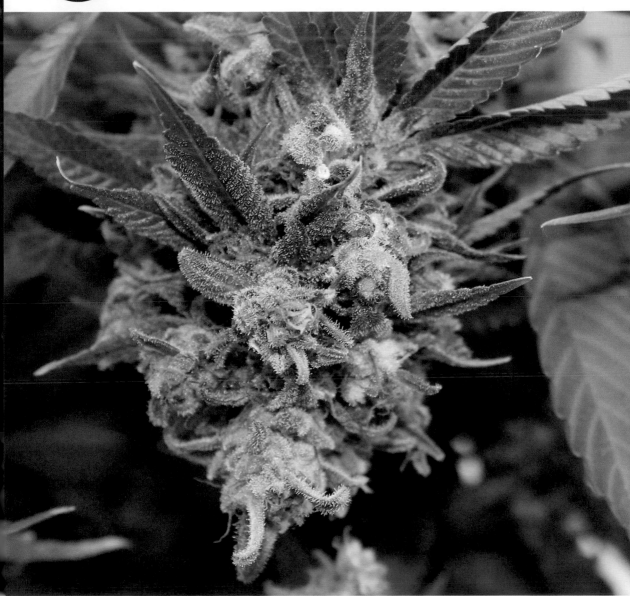
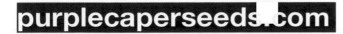
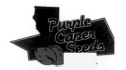

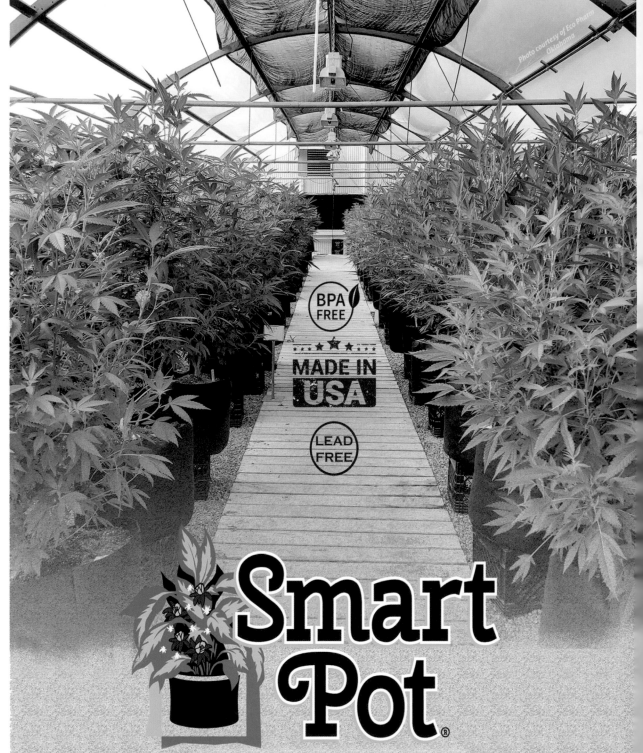

Photo courtesy of Eco Pharm
Oklahoma

Smart Pot®

Patented Aeration Container

Performance Gardening® *with Performance Profits*

www.SmartPots.com

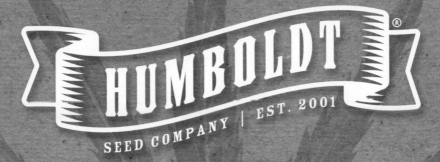
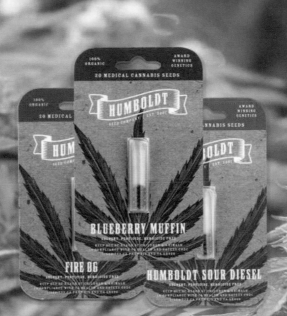

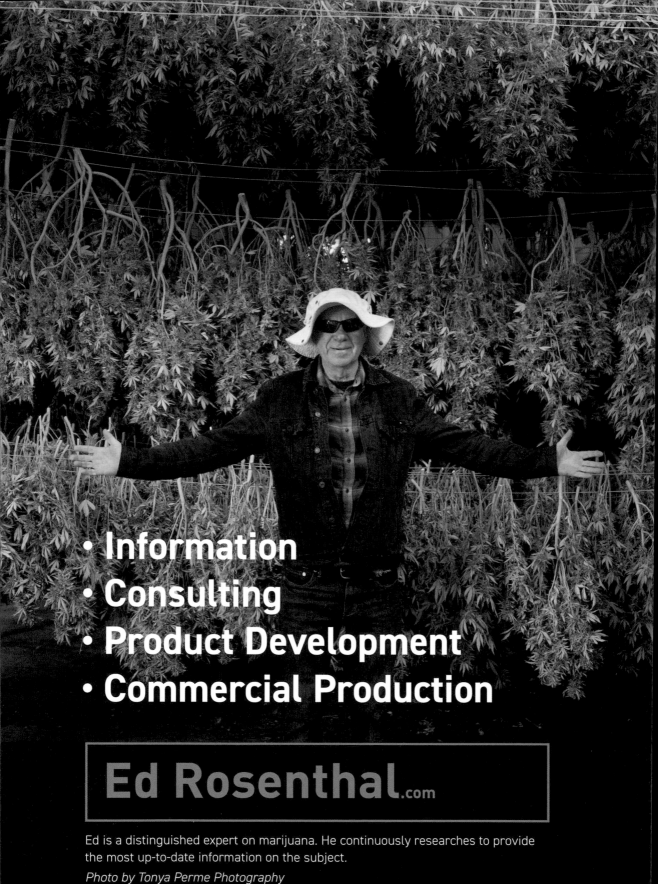

- **Information**
- **Consulting**
- **Product Development**
- **Commercial Production**

Ed Rosenthal.com

Ed is a distinguished expert on marijuana. He continuously researches to provide the most up-to-date information on the subject.

Photo by Tonya Perme Photography

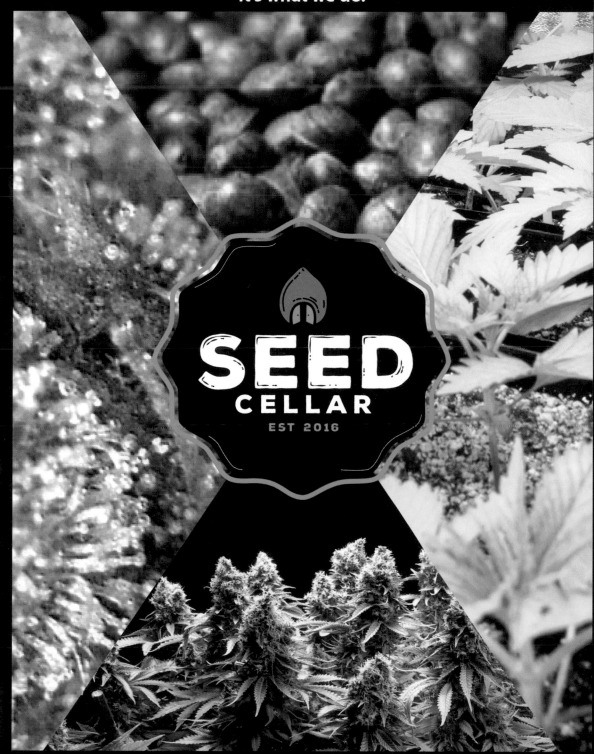

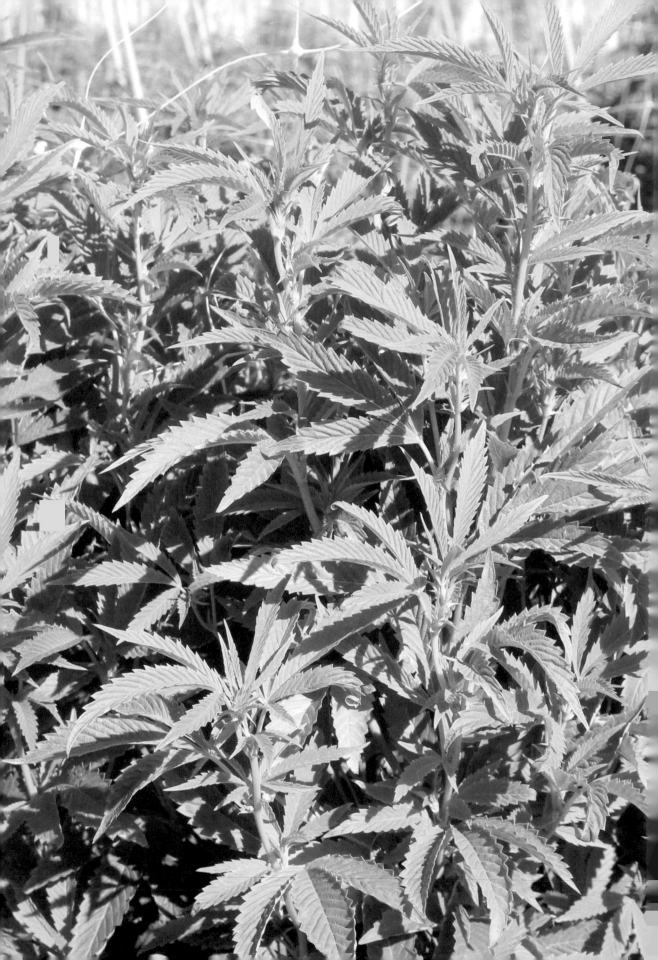